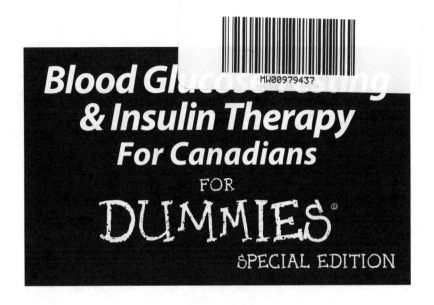

Blood Glucose Testing & Insulin Therapy
For Canadians

FOR
DUMMIES®

SPECIAL EDITION

by Ian Blumer, MD, FRCPC
Alan L. Rubin, MD

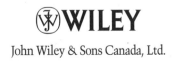

John Wiley & Sons Canada, Ltd.

Blood Glucose Testing & Insulin Therapy For Canadians For Dummies®

Published by
John Wiley & Sons Canada, Ltd.
6045 Freemont Blvd.
Mississauga, ON L5R 4J3
www.wiley.com

ISBN: 978-1-118-01111-9

Printed in Canada

1 2 3 4 5 PC 14 13 12 11 10

For details on how to create a custom book for your company or organization, or for more information on John Wiley & Sons Canada custom publishing programs, please call 416-646-7992 or email publishingbyobjectives@wiley.com.

For general information on John Wiley & Sons Canada, Ltd., including all books published by Wiley Publishing Inc., please call our distribution centre at 1-800-567-4797. For reseller information, including discounts and premium sales, please call our sales department at 416-646-7992. For press review copies, author interviews, or other publicity information, please contact our publicity department, Tel. 416-646-4582, Fax 416-236-4448.

This book is an edited excerpt of *Diabetes For Canadians For Dummies*, Second Edition. Advertising materials in this special edition have been supplied by Abbott Diabetes Care. The publisher and authors do not recommend or promote a specific method, treatment, or product.

WILEY

About the Authors

Ian Blumer, MD, FRCPC, is a diabetes specialist in the Greater Toronto Area of Ontario. He has a teaching appointment with the University of Toronto, is the medical advisor to the adult program of the Charles H. Best Diabetes Centre in Whitby, Ontario, and is actively involved in diabetes research. An enthusiastic lecturer, he has spoken about diabetes to numerous professional and lay audiences and has appeared regularly in the Canadian media.

Dr. Blumer is a member of the Clinical and Scientific Section of the Canadian Diabetes Association (CDA), where he currently serves as Chair of the Dissemination and Implementation Committee for the 2008 CDA Clinical Practice Guidelines. He is also a member of the American Diabetes Association, and the European Association for the Study of Diabetes.

Dr. Blumer is the co-author of *Diabetes Cookbook For Canadians For Dummies, Diabetes For Canadians For Dummies, Understanding Prescription Drugs For Canadians For Dummies,* and *Celiac Disease For Dummies.* He is also the author of *What Your Doctor Really Thinks.* His Web site (www.ourdiabetes.com) offers practical advice on how to manage diabetes. Ian welcomes your comments about this book at diabetes@ianblumer.com.

Alan L. Rubin, MD, is one of America's foremost experts on diabetes. He is a professional member of the American Diabetes Association and the Endocrine Society and has been in private practice specializing in diabetes and thyroid disease for more than 30 years. Dr. Rubin was Assistant Clinical Professor of Medicine at University of California Medical Center in San Francisco for 20 years. He has spoken about diabetes to professional medical audiences and non-medical audiences around the world. He has been a consultant to many pharmaceutical companies and companies that make diabetes products.

Dr. Rubin was one of the first specialists in his field to recognize the significance of patient self-testing of blood glucose, the major advance in diabetes care since the advent of insulin. As a result, he has been on numerous radio and television programs, talking about the cause, the prevention, and the treatment of diabetes and its complications.

Since publishing *Diabetes For Dummies,* Dr. Rubin has had four other bestselling *For Dummies* books — *Diabetes Cookbook For Dummies, Thyroid For Dummies, High Blood Pressure For Dummies,* and *Type 1 Diabetes For Dummies* — all published by Wiley.

Publisher's Acknowledgements

We're proud of this book; please send us your comments at
http://dummies.custhelp.com.

Some of the people who helped bring this book to market include the following:

Acquisitions and Editorial

Acquiring Editor: Robert Hickey

Manager, Custom Publications:
Christiane Coté

Production Editor: Pamela Vokey

Editorial Assistant: Katie Wolsley

Composition Services

Vice-President, Publishing Services:
Karen Bryan

Layout and Graphics: Pat Loi

Proofreader: Heather Ball

John Wiley & Sons Canada, Ltd.

Deborah Barton, Vice President and Director of Operations

Karen Bryan, Vice-President, Publishing Services

Jennifer Smith, Vice-President and Publisher, Professional & Trade Division

Alison Maclean, Managing Editor

Publishing and Editorial for Consumer Dummies

Diane Graves Steele, Vice President and Publisher, Consumer Dummies

Kristin Ferguson-Wagstaffe, Product Development Director, Consumer Dummies

Ensley Eikenburg, Associate Publisher, Travel

Kelly Regan, Editorial Director, Travel

Composition Services

Debbie Stailey, Director of Composition Services

Table of Contents

Chapter 4: Ten Ways to Stay Healthy and Avoid Complications 97

Chapter 5: Ten Frequently Asked Questions 107

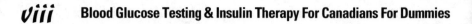

Introduction

● ●

*I*f you have diabetes, you're not alone; you're part of a group that's growing every day. In 1985 there were 30 million people with diabetes in the world. By 2000 that number had risen to 150 million. By the year 2025 it's estimated that 380 million people will have diabetes. If you're like us, these numbers sound alarming but are so large they're hard to relate to. So, looking closer to home, a recent study found that from 1995 to 2005 the number of people in Ontario living with diabetes doubled, reaching 9 percent of the population, or 827,000 individuals. (It is quite likely that similar figures are present elsewhere in Canada, too.) Nine percent! Next time you're at a hockey game, look around the stands and just imagine that nearly one in ten people in the arena have diabetes.

Although there may never be a good time to have diabetes, it's far better to have it now than 100 years ago, when almost no therapy was available. Until insulin was discovered in the 1920s, little could be done to help people with diabetes. Nowadays, however, many types of medicines — including many different types of insulin — are available to help keep your blood glucose levels in check. And recent discoveries will lead to additional, helpful medication options becoming available over the next few years. As Ian likes to say, it was about time that diabetes specialists were given more tools; we were getting very jealous of cardiologists who seemed to be getting all the neat drugs. Nowadays virtually anyone with diabetes can have excellent blood glucose control. It may not always be easy to achieve, but it can be achieved and must be achieved if you are going to keep healthy.

About This Book

This book, excerpted from *Diabetes For Canadians For Dummies*, is intended to help people living with insulin-treated diabetes learn about monitoring blood glucose levels, dealing with blood glucose emergencies, and using insulin effectively so that they can achieve and maintain good health. You don't have to read it cover to cover, but if you know nothing about blood glucose or insulin, doing so may be a good approach. (To learn about the whole breadth of diabetes, including the ins and outs of non-insulin therapies, we unabashedly refer you to the full text version of *Diabetes For Canadians For Dummies.*)

This book looks at some of the special issues that Canadians with insulin-treated diabetes have to face (like Ian's patient who returned to his car one February morning after his son's hockey practice, only to find his insulin frozen solid!) and uses the most recent Canadian Diabetes Association recommendations *(2008 Clinical Practice Guidelines for the Prevention and Management of Diabetes in Canada).* These guidelines are of such high quality that they're referred to and used around the world. (You can find the guidelines online at www.diabetes. ca/for-professionals/resources/2008-cpg).

Conventions Used in This Book

Diabetes, as you know, is associated with sugar problems. But sugars come in many types, so doctors avoid using the words *sugar* and *glucose* interchangeably. In this book, we use the word *glucose* rather than *sugar* (unless we're talking about things such as table sugar or sweets you have in your diet). As well, because it gets to be redundant to keep adding mmol/L (which is short for millimoles per litre) after every blood glucose value to which we refer, you can safely assume that when we say, for example, that a fasting blood glucose of 7 (or higher) is indicative of diabetes, we mean 7.0 mmol/L.

What You Don't Have to Read

We hope you'll enjoy reading everything in this book; however, throughout the book, you'll find shaded areas, which are called sidebars, that contain material that's interesting but not essential. We hereby give you permission to skip them if the material they cover is of no particular interest to you. You'll still understand everything else.

In addition, we've noted some paragraphs that have a more technical nature with the Technical Stuff icon (see the section "Icons Used in This Book," later in this Introduction for more information on icons). Although these paragraphs deepen your knowledge of diabetes, you can still understand the text without reading them. Our feelings won't get hurt if you don't read these paragraphs, but these technical tidbits may come in handy during a high-stakes trivia game, or at the very least can make you sound pretty smart in front of your doctor.

Icons Used in This Book

Throughout this book, on the left-hand side of the page, are little pictures, called *icons*. The icons tell you what you must know, what you should know, and what you might find interesting but can live without:

This icon indicates a story about one of our patients. (The names and other identifiers have been changed to maintain confidentiality.)

This icon gives you technical information or terminology that may be helpful, but not necessary, to your understanding of the topic.

When you see this icon, it means the information is critical and is not to be missed.

This icon points out when you should contact your health care team (for example, if your blood glucose control is in need of improving or if you need a particular test done). Your health care team includes your family doctor, your diabetes specialist, your diabetes nurse educator, your dietitian, your eye doctor (optometrist or ophthalmologist), your pharmacist, and, when necessary, other specialists (such as a podiatrist, dentist, cardiologist, kidney specialist, neurologist, emergency room physician, and so forth). We'll let you know which member of your team you should contact. (Incidentally, the most important member of your health care team is *you.*)

This icon is used when we share a practical, time-saving piece of advice, sometimes providing some additional detail on an important point.

Chapter 1

Handling Low and High Blood Glucose Emergencies

*B*lood glucose control in diabetes involves two separate issues. On the one hand, you have your long-term goal of maintaining good glucose levels to feel well and to avoid damaging your body as time goes by. On the other hand, you may face situations when your blood glucose control suddenly deteriorates and requires urgent attention. In this chapter we discuss those circumstances that require immediate action.

With the exception of *mild hypoglycemia* (low blood glucose that you can manage yourself), you should treat all the issues we look at in this chapter as medical emergencies. Don't try to treat these complications by yourself. You or the person assisting you should contact your health care team or, if necessary, call 911. In this chapter we discuss when and whom to call.

Understanding Hypoglycemia (Low Blood Glucose)

Hypoglycemia is a blood glucose level below normal. That much is straightforward. The problem is defining precisely how low a normal blood glucose can be. This is a subject of some controversy in the medical community, with widely varying numbers used. However, the Canadian Diabetes Association 2008 Clinical Practice Guidelines (upon which this book is based) consider hypoglycemia to be a blood glucose level of less than 4.0 mmol/L (*if* you are taking certain medications like insulin injections).

Your body doesn't function well when you have too little glucose in your blood. Your brain needs glucose to allow you to think properly, and your muscles need the energy that glucose provides in much the same way that your car needs gasoline to run. As we discover in this chapter, diabetes in and of itself does not cause hypoglycemia; rather, certain *treatments* for diabetes can cause hypoglycemia.

Having diabetes isn't fair. It's unfair to get it. It's unfair to develop complications. And it's especially unfair that those people with diabetes who try the hardest to stay healthy are the most prone to getting hypoglycemia. If you have poorly controlled glucose levels with values running between 15 and 20, you may not feel great, but you are highly unlikely ever to run into significant problems with hypoglycemia. But if you look after yourself meticulously and keep your blood glucose levels in the 4 to 8 range, you are at much greater risk of having hypoglycemia. Fortunately, it is possible to have excellent control and, at the same time, to minimize the risk of getting hypoglycemia. It ain't easy, but it is doable. We discuss how to do it later in this section.

Not every person develops symptoms of hypoglycemia at the same level of blood glucose. Some people notice it at blood glucose levels of 3.8, others only when their blood glucose level is between 2 and 3. Moreover, a person might notice it on one occasion when his or her blood glucose level is below 3.6 and that *same* person might not notice it on another occasion until it's below 3.2. You also need to remember that glucose meters aren't perfect. You may have already discovered that you can check your reading seconds apart and find discrepancies of up to 15 percent. That doesn't mean your blood glucose level changed that much in that brief interval. It simply means the machines aren't precision instruments. (But if your machine gives readings — checked moments apart — that differ by *more than* 15 percent, have your device checked to make sure it isn't malfunctioning.)

Looking at the symptoms of hypoglycemia

Doctors traditionally divide the symptoms of hypoglycemia into two major categories:

- ✔ **Autonomic symptoms** are symptoms (such as tremors and palpitations, as we discuss below) that are due to the effects of the hormones (especially epinephrine, also called adrenaline) that your body sends out to counter low blood glucose. They are called autonomic symptoms because they arise from the autonomic (automatic in a sense) part of your nervous system.

- ✔ **Neuroglycopenic symptoms** are symptoms (such as confusion and disorientation, as we discuss later in this section) that are due to your brain not receiving enough glucose. Neuroglycopenic is derived from neuro (referring to the nervous system), glyco (glucose), and penic (insufficient).

The severity of hypoglycemia can be classified as

- ✔ **Mild:** Autonomic symptoms are present and you're able to treat yourself.

- ✔ **Moderate:** Autonomic and neuroglycopenic symptoms are present and you're able to treat yourself.

- ✔ **Severe:** Hypoglycemia is bad enough that you require someone else to assist you. Unconsciousness may occur. (With severe hypoglycemia, the blood glucose is typically less than 2.8 mmol/L.)

The main reason to know this classification is so that you and your health care providers are sure to be on the same page. Otherwise, there could be miscommunication and inappropriate advice given to you. For example, if you are on insulin and you tell your doctor you had a "severe low," your doctor may interpret this as per the above definition and give you advice — like substantially reducing your insulin dose — based on that. But if by "severe low" you *actually* meant you felt really, really crummy, but in fact your blood glucose was only slightly decreased (say, 3.6 mmol/L) and you were able to easily treat yourself by drinking a glass of pop, then you would likely receive very different advice from your doctor.

If you take medicines (such as insulin) that can cause hypoglycemia, for your own safety it would be very wise to wear a medical alert bracelet or necklace. At the very least (though certainly not as good), carry some form of identification in your purse or wallet noting that you have diabetes. You may never need them, but it's a good idea to be prepared just in case. We've had more than one patient who has received necessary emergency care (for hypoglycemia) that might not have been given if a passerby had not seen the person's medical alert and instead mistakenly assumed he was drunk. (We've also had patients who were hypoglycemic and, as a result, driving erratically, but who might have been arrested for suspected drunk driving if the police officer hadn't noticed the person's medical alert stating that they had diabetes.)

Most people with diabetes go their entire lives without ever experiencing even a single episode of *severe* hypoglycemia. The vast majority of the time, if you are experiencing hypoglycemia, the early warning autonomic symptoms kick in and allow you to quickly rectify the problem.

A close call

Ian had a young adult patient with insulin-treated diabetes who experienced an episode of severe hypoglycemia whilst driving. The hypoglycemia caused the man to be driving erratically to the point that he drove off the road and came to a stop on an embankment. Fortunately, no one was hurt. A police officer saw what had transpired and, thinking the man was drunk or high on drugs, was about to put handcuffs on him and arrest him, but the officer caught sight of the man's medical alert bracelet stating that he had diabetes. The officer helped treat Ian's patient, who quickly recovered. Goodness knows what might have happened had the patient not been wearing the medical alert.

Autonomic symptoms

Autonomic symptoms are your best friends. They're your warning system alerting you to a problem of low blood glucose and demanding that you attend to it before it progresses to the more dangerous neuroglycopenic stage (which we discuss shortly).

Autonomic symptoms are

- ✔ Anxiety
- ✔ Hunger
- ✔ Nausea
- ✔ Palpitations (noticing a rapid or excessively forceful heartbeat)
- ✔ Sweating
- ✔ Tingling (numbness)
- ✔ Trembling (shaking of your body, especially the hands)

As you look through the above list, you may realize you've had some or all of these symptoms at various times in your life, even if you've never been on medicine that could cause low blood glucose. The reason: These symptoms can occur in *any* situation where epinephrine levels are high, and that includes so-called fight-or-flight situations where you're under extreme stress. (Examples are if you're about to write a difficult exam, about to have a job interview, or are writing a book on diabetes and your editor calls you to let you know your manuscript is due . . . yesterday. Eeek.)

Because symptoms such as sweating or palpitations, which can indicate hypoglycemia, can also occur in situations such as stress, where your blood glucose level may actually be perfectly normal, you should conclude that you have hypoglycemia only if you have demonstrated a low blood glucose level on your glucose meter.

Shortly after you begin therapy for high blood glucose, you may find that you're experiencing autonomic symptoms, suggesting you have hypoglycemia even though your blood glucose levels may not be low. This is perfectly normal — it will take a few days for your body to become accustomed to having normal blood glucose levels, at which point your symptoms will resolve (that is, they'll go away).

If you are on medications such as insulin or certain oral blood-glucose lowering drugs (especially a drug called glyburide), it's quite possible that you recall having had at least one episode where your hands started to shake, you became sweaty and hungry, and you recognized that something wasn't quite right. You probably reached for your glucose meter, checked your blood glucose level, and found it to be somewhere in the low 3s. You likely took some sugar candies or a glass of juice or pop and felt better within a few minutes. Congratulations: You successfully diagnosed, treated, and cured your first patient. Feel free to write the rest of this chapter. Oh, never mind, we'll do it.

Neuroglycopenic symptoms

Neuroglycopenic symptoms are much more of a problem. These symptoms are most definitely not your friends — quite the opposite. Whereas autonomic symptoms alert you to a problem, neuroglycopenic symptoms often interfere with your ability to recognize and deal with hypoglycemia. By the time these symptoms develop, your blood glucose level is usually profoundly low and has become a true emergency. These symptoms include

- Confusion
- Difficulty concentrating
- Difficulty speaking
- Dizziness
- Drowsiness
- Headache
- Loss of consciousness (coma)
- Seizures
- Tiredness
- Vision changes (such as double vision or loss of vision)
- Weakness

People lose their ability to think clearly when they become hypoglycemic. They make simple errors, and other people often assume that they're drunk. Suffice it to say, if Albert Einstein were having an episode of hypoglycemia, he may have ended up mistakenly deciding E = mc. And if similarly affected, Wayne Gretzky would have been the not-quite-as-Great One. Fortunately, adult brains have an amazing capacity to put up with insults like hypoglycemia, and long-term damage to the brain from low blood glucose almost never occurs. Because the brains of infants and young children are more sensitive to injury, however, it's especially important to avoid severe hypoglycemia in this age group (we define severe hypoglycemia earlier in this section).

Considering the causes of hypoglycemia

Hypoglycemia doesn't cause diabetes. Now, in another attempt to dispel popular misconceptions, we wish to hereby announce that diabetes doesn't cause hypoglycemia. Remember, you read it here first. Certain medicines used to *treat* diabetes can cause hypoglycemia, but hypoglycemia is not caused by diabetes in and of itself. Indeed, if you have diabetes and are being treated purely with lifestyle measures (nutrition and exercise therapy), you will *never* experience hypoglycemia.

Hypoglycemia is always unintended. Ideally, your blood glucose levels would always be normal — never high, never low. Unfortunately, we seldom have that degree of success with our imperfect therapies. A number of the medicines we use to prevent blood glucose levels from being too high have the potential to drop them too low. These medicines are

✔ **Insulin:** Unlike insulin made by your pancreas, insulin you inject does not have the ability to turn itself off the instant you no longer need it. An injection of insulin will help to reduce your blood glucose level, but it also has the potential to drop your level excessively. This drop is called an *insulin reaction*. (You may have heard the term insulin shock used in reference to particularly bad insulin reactions. Insulin shock is not a scientific term, however, and can be misleading. Indeed, we would prefer the term never be used. Accordingly, we won't be using it beyond this brief explanation.) We discuss insulin therapy in detail in Chapter 3.

✔ **Sulfonylurea medicine:** Medicines from this family have the potential to cause low blood glucose. This is particularly true of glyburide.

✔ **Meglitinides:** Never do we, as diabetes specialists, consider ourselves luckier than when we attend conferences where these medicines are discussed. Oh no, not just because they're important drugs to know about. No. We consider ourselves fortunate because at these conferences we learn how to pronounce them! Don't worry; no one uses these names anyhow. Doctors pretty well just use the trade names (GlucoNorm, Starlix) for drugs currently available within this group. These drugs, like sulfonylureas, make the pancreas release extra insulin and have the potential to cause hypoglycemia.

Although these medicines can cause hypoglycemia, you can improve the odds that they won't by taking certain precautions. We discuss these precautions later in this chapter.

Treating hypoglycemia

The vast majority of episodes of hypoglycemia are mild (or moderate; see the definitions of these terms earlier in this section) and you will be able to deal with them easily. Nonetheless — particularly if you have type 1 diabetes — severe episodes can and do occur, so it is best for you and your loved ones (and friends, workmates, and so on) to know what to do in the event that this happens to you. In this section we look at these important issues.

Treating mild and moderate hypoglycemia

If you find that your blood glucose level is low, then you must ingest some sugar to restore your level to normal. The Canadian Diabetes Association (CDA) recommends that if you have mild to moderate hypoglycemia (that is, you are still awake and aware enough to take things by mouth), you should take the following steps:

✔ **Step One:** Eat or drink 15 grams of a fast-acting carbohy-drate such as

- Four 4-gram tablets (for example, four Dex4 tablets, which works out to 16 grams of glucose, but that's similar enough to 15 grams that your body won't notice the difference)
- 175 mL (¾ cup) of juice or regular (not diet or sugar-free) pop (but see the tip following this list)
- 15 mL (3 tsp) honey
- 15 mL (3 tsp) table sugar dissolved in water

✔ **Step Two:** Wait 15 minutes, and then retest your blood. If your blood glucose level is still less than 4 mmol/L, ingest another 15 grams of carbohydrate.

✔ **Step Three:** If your next meal is more than one hour away, or you are going to be physically active, eat a snack, such as half a sandwich or cheese and crackers. The snack should contain 15 grams of carbohydrate and a source of protein.

Despite what most people think (and do), orange juice (or milk or, especially, glucose gel) is not as effective as products like Dextrosol because it raises glucose levels and relieves you of symptoms more slowly. Nonetheless, if you have some O.J. and it's handier than an alternative, it will work.

Because acarbose (Glucobay) slows down absorption of sucrose, if you are taking this medicine and you develop hypoglycemia, you should be treated with glucose (such as Dextrosol), not sucrose (such as fruit juice).

If you are hypoglycemic and you're about to eat a meal, you should *first* treat your hypoglycemia with a fast-acting carbo-hydrate as described above. This will ensure that your blood glucose is brought up rapidly.

Because the symptoms of hypoglycemia are so unpleasant and because hypoglycemia is understandably scary, you may find yourself taking candy after candy until you feel better without actually giving time for the first treatment to take effect. Then, when all that sugar you have just ingested gets absorbed into your system, you may find that your glucose level is up into the teens. It is best, therefore, to give the first treatment time (as described earlier) to work before you take another.

Dealing with severe hypoglycemia

Because your mental state may be impaired when you have hypoglycemia, you need to make sure that your friends or relatives know in advance what hypoglycemia is and what to do about it. Having people around you who are aware is especially important if your hypoglycemia is so bad that you are unconscious or nearly so, in which case you will be unable to swallow properly. In this circumstance, people should *not* try to feed you, because you could choke. Instead, your helper should administer glucagon (see the "Using glucagon" section) to you, and also should call 911 to summon an ambulance. If you experience milder hypoglycemia, where you are alert but somewhat confused and unable to obtain an appropriate sugar source, then your helper simply needs to find one for you and help you to ingest it.

Inform people about your diabetes and about how to recognize hypoglycemia. Let them know where you store your emergency supplies (such as the glucose tablets you use to treat hypoglycemia). Don't keep your diabetes a secret. The people close to you will be glad to know how to help you.

Using glucagon

Glucagon is available by prescription in a package called a *glucagon kit*. This kit includes a syringe and 1 mg of glucagon, one of the major hormones that raises glucose, which your helper should inject into your leg muscle (the buttock and arm can also be used). (Half that dose — that is, 0.5 mg — should be used if you are treating a child 5 years of age or less.) The injection of glucagon raises the blood glucose, and within 15 to 20 minutes you will likely become fully alert.

If you have just experienced a severe episode of hypoglycemia and you required an injection of glucagon, then once you have fully come around and are again able to swallow properly, you should consume some quick-acting hypoglycemia treatment (see the list earlier in this section) followed by food to help prevent your redeveloping hypoglycemia as the glucagon wears off.

Some people are, understandably, just too nervous or too intimidated to take it upon themselves to administer glucagon. In that case, they should just call an ambulance.

Remember that when you pick up the glucagon kit from the pharmacy, the person who is most likely to be giving it should go with you. The pharmacist *must* sit down and explain to both of you how it is given.

Like most medicines, glucagon has an expiration date after which it may not work sufficiently well. For this reason, as soon as you pick up your glucagon kit, find out when it will expire and mark on your calendar a few weeks in advance of the expiration date a reminder for you to pick up a new kit.

If you live, work, or play in an area where emergency health care services are more than just minutes away, it's especially important for you to have a glucagon kit. Do you snowmobile? Hunt? Hike? Boat? Do you live in a remote area? Does your job take you into the bush? All of these situations would warrant having a supply of glucagon readily available. Keep in mind the Boy Scouts' motto: Be prepared.

If you are the parent of a young child, you likely know all too well the phrases "I'm not hungry" or "I don't want to eat." These typically relatively harmless situations, however, take on a potentially much more serious meaning if your child has diabetes and is receiving insulin therapy. In this case, without food, your child will be at risk of hypoglycemia. If your child is receiving insulin, refuses food, and then develops mild hypoglycemia (or is about to), you can give her mini-doses of glucagon. The glucagon will help ward off or reverse hypoglycemia. We recommend you speak to your child's diabetes specialist or diabetes educator to find out more information on when you would use glucagon and the doses to administer.

Notifying your health team

If you have experienced severe hypoglycemia — even if you quickly recovered — it's crucial that you notify your family physician, your diabetes specialist, or your diabetes educator(s) so that they can make appropriate adjustments to your therapy to lessen the likelihood of your having another severe attack. If you're feeling well and have fully recovered from the episode, you don't have to call your health care team right away, but it would be wise to get in touch with them within a day or two.

Preventing hypoglycemia

Not everyone with diabetes experiences hypoglycemia. As we discuss earlier in this chapter, if your treatment is lifestyle therapy alone, you won't have low blood glucose. However, most people with diabetes at some point will require use of medicines (such as insulin or a sulfonylurea) that will put them at risk of hypoglycemia.

Although no foolproof way to avoid hypoglycemia exists, you can follow the following techniques:

- **Don't miss or delay meals:** Because pills and insulin that are used to reduce blood glucose do not have the good sense to know exactly when to stop working, like the famous battery-operated bunny, they sometimes tend to keep going and going. (Precisely how long depends on the particular type of insulin that you are using; we discuss this in Chapter 3.) That would be fine if your glucose level is still high, but not so fine if your level has come back to normal, as it most likely will have by the time your next meal rolls around. If your meal is unduly delayed, the medicine may pull your glucose level down too low.

- **Plan your exercise:** Exercise is an essential component of your diabetes therapy (particularly if you have type 2 diabetes). But it's important for you to be aware that exercise accelerates the rate at which glucose moves from the blood into muscle (where it's used as fuel) and, thus, can cause you to have hypoglycemia. By all means *do* exercise; however, if you know from experience that when you perform a certain type or amount of exercise you develop hypoglycemia, speak to your diabetes educator or physician about how to adjust your medicines or diet to reduce the risk of developing low blood glucose. Often the solution is something as simple as having a small snack before (or even while) you work out. The worst thing is to have hypoglycemia every time you exercise; we can't imagine a stronger disincentive to exercising than that!

✔ **Have a bedtime snack:** Eating a bedtime snack is not necessary for most people with diabetes unless you're taking evening doses of insulin and your bedtime blood glucose level is less than 7 mmol/L, in which case a bedtime snack containing at least 15 grams of carbohydrate and 15 grams of protein will help you avoid having a low reading overnight. If you find that going to bed with a higher glucose level does not prevent overnight lows, then you should take a snack even if your bedtime reading is higher than 7 mmol/L. (As we discuss in Chapter 3, if you are on insulin it's a good idea to periodically test your blood glucose level at about 3 a.m. to make sure it is not going low overnight without your having recognized it.)

✔ **Change your oral hypoglycemic agent or insulin therapy if necessary:** If your current treatments are resulting in hypoglycemia, speak to your physician about whether you would benefit from a change to your diabetes medicines. This may be something as simple as a small dose change or as major as changing to a different medicine altogether.

✔ **Pay close attention to your symptoms of hypoglycemia:** By knowing what symptoms you typically get when you have hypoglycemia, you will be able to recognize hypoglycemia faster and treat it earlier.

✔ **Avoid (or minimize) the use of other drugs that can cause hypoglycemia:** Several drugs (not specifically being used to treat your diabetes) that you may take from time to time have the potential to lower your blood glucose levels. These drugs include alcohol and *high* doses of Aspirin (ASA). If you are experiencing hypoglycemia, make sure you review *all* your medicines with your doctor to see if you should make some changes.

✔ **Set higher blood glucose targets:** For some people, despite their (and their diabetes team's) best efforts, recurring hypoglycemia is still a problem. (This is rarely the case unless you have type 1 diabetes.) In this situation, the only way to avoid repeated episodes of hypoglycemia may be to set blood glucose goals somewhat higher than the CDA target (see Chapter 2). We recommend you discuss with your doctor and your diabetes educator what your specific targets should be.

> ✔ **Wear a continuous glucose monitoring system (CGMS):**
> These recently developed devices continuously measure your (interstitial fluid) glucose level and alarm you if your level is heading too low. They are particularly suited to people with type 1 diabetes on insulin pump therapy. We discuss continuous glucose monitoring systems in detail in Chapter 2.

If you are on intensified insulin therapy (see Chapter 3), episodes of hypoglycemia are inevitable. Ian has found that, as a very rough rule of thumb, to achieve excellent overall blood glucose control, you can expect to have *mild* hypoglycemia about two to three times per week. More frequent hypoglycemia may put you at undue risk of severe hypoglycemia. On the other hand, if you are on intensified insulin therapy and you are *never* experiencing episodes of hypoglycemia, your average blood glucose level is probably too high.

We discuss additional tips for people on insulin therapy in Chapter 3.

Coping with hypoglycemia unawareness

Hypoglycemia unawareness is a condition in which you lose your ability to recognize when your blood glucose level has fallen below normal. Samantha, one of Ian's patients, had this condition.

Samantha was 28 years old. She had developed diabetes when she was only 5 years of age. Samantha was a highly motivated patient and was monitoring her blood glucose levels many times per day. With aggressive use of insulin, nutrition therapy, and exercise, she was able to keep her glucose readings generally between 3.8 and 7.6. Recently, while she was at work, her boss had found her staring vacantly into space. He was able to get her to drink some juice and she quickly came around, but the next day the same thing happened again. Two days later, her husband awakened to find Samantha soaking wet in bed beside him. He couldn't awaken her. He tested her blood and found her glucose level to be 1.8. He gave her an injection of glucagon (see earlier for a discussion about glucagon) and over the next 15 minutes she gradually awakened. Later that day, she went to see Ian in the office, her therapy was adjusted, and soon thereafter she was able to once again recognize when her blood glucose levels were too low.

A condition like Samantha's can occur for several reasons:

- **Repeated hypoglycemia:** If you have been experiencing frequent hypoglycemia — even if mild — your autonomic warning system (such as sweating and palpitations; see the "Autonomic symptoms" section, earlier in this chapter) may start to fail and the first clue that you have low blood glucose can be when you are confused and unable to look after yourself. The best way to correct this is, *under your diabetes specialist's guidance,* to somewhat reduce your insulin doses to avoid any and all hypoglycemia for a few weeks, at which point your doses can typically be again increased with restoration of hypoglycemia awareness.

- **Longstanding diabetes:** Occasionally, if you have had diabetes for a very long time (generally speaking, we are talking decades), your autonomic warning system may fail and, as in Samantha's situation, the first clue there is a problem may be when you become confused. Setting higher blood glucose targets may be required. Also, using a CGMS (see the "Preventing hypoglycemia" section and Chapter 2) may be helpful.

- **Other drugs impairing your ability to recognize hypoglycemia:** Several drugs can interfere with your body's ability to produce autonomic symptoms. Such drugs include beta blockers (such as atenolol), which are often used to treat heart disease and high blood pressure. If a medication is responsible, your physician (in consultation with you) will need to determine if another medication may be substituted. Another drug that you may have passing acquaintance with is alcohol, which, if used in sufficient quantities that impair your alertness, can blunt your ability to recognize when you're hypoglycemic.

Dealing with Ketoacidosis

If you have type 1 diabetes, you're at risk for developing a dangerous, temporary condition called *diabetic ketoacidosis* (typically just called ketoacidosis or by its abbreviated form, DKA) in which your blood glucose level is high (typically above 14) *and* you have excess quantities of a type of acid called *ketones* in the blood. High blood glucose *without* the presence of ketones does not indicate DKA. (Though, of course, it might indicate your glucose control is pretty crummy, but that is a different story.)

Ketoacidosis requires urgent attention because, if severe, it can be life-threatening. Occasionally, the first clue that you have type 1 diabetes is when you become ill with ketoacidosis. More commonly, DKA occurs after you already know that you have the disease.

Exploring how ketoacidosis develops

The main source of energy for your muscles is glucose. And for glucose to be used properly you must have sufficient insulin in your body. If you have type 1 diabetes, you lack the ability to produce insulin and, thus, you need to give it to yourself by injection.

But what happens if your body requires more insulin than you are giving? Several things can happen:

- ✔ Your blood glucose levels will climb (because the glucose can't get into your cells without sufficient insulin to help it).
- ✔ Your body will start to break down fat (and muscle) because it can't use glucose as a fuel.
- ✔ As fat tissue breaks down, it releases acids (ketones) into the bloodstream.

The result is that you develop ketoacidosis.

Investigating the symptoms of ketoacidosis

These are the symptoms of ketoacidosis:

- ✔ **Extreme tiredness and drowsiness:** If your DKA is mild, your tiredness may also be mild, but as your DKA worsens you will feel increasingly drowsy, and if your DKA becomes severe you can lose consciousness.

✓ **Fruity breath:** The presence of ketones in your system gives your breath a fruity, not unpleasant, odour. Most people with DKA do not notice it even though it might be apparent to bystanders.

✓ **Nausea, vomiting, and abdominal pain:** It is noteworthy that many people with diabetes — and many doctors also, by the way — mistakenly attribute these symptoms to stomach flu *(gastroenteritis)* even when they are due to DKA. (Of course you *may* simply have the flu, but a doctor should come to this conclusion only after DKA has been excluded.)

✓ **Rapid breathing:** You experience rapid breathing when your blood is so acidic that your body tries to compensate by ridding itself of acids through the lungs.

The Canadian Diabetes Association recommends that people with type 1 diabetes test for ketones

✓ During periods of acute illness when elevated blood glucose readings are present

✓ When before-meal blood glucose readings are above 14 mmol/L

✓ When symptoms of DKA (see earlier) are present

Ketoacidosis occurs rarely in type 2 diabetes. Nonetheless, if you have type 2 diabetes and you develop typical symptoms of DKA, it would be a good idea to check for ketones.

Although ketones can be tested in the urine (by urinating on test strips; several companies make these strips), it is preferable to test for them in the blood (with use of the Precision Xtra blood glucose and blood ketone testing meter; this is the only blood ketone tester available in Canada).

If you notice that you have symptoms of ketoacidosis and you test your blood ketone level and find it to be elevated (0.6 mmol/L or higher), in most cases the safest and best thing to do is to go to the closest emergency department. However, if your symptoms are mild and you are fortunate enough to be working with a diabetes educator who is trained — and empowered — to deal with DKA (and is immediately available), you can first contact her or him for detailed advice.

Understanding the causes of ketoacidosis

Ketoacidosis is caused by a *relative* lack of insulin. And no, this does not mean that it is caused by your first cousin Sally not having enough insulin. (Though perhaps she doesn't. We wouldn't know.) When we say *relative* lack of insulin, we mean that the amount of insulin in your body — no matter how much there is — is not enough for your body's needs. It follows, then, that DKA will develop in one of two general circumstances:

- ✔ **You are missing insulin doses:** If you have type 1 diabetes, your pancreas is unable to manufacture insulin, so you must give yourself insulin. If you miss doses, your body quickly detects this and your metabolism will promptly suffer. (See Chapter 3 for a detailed discussion of insulin.) The occasional missed dose of rapid-acting or regular insulin isn't likely to harm you, but if you miss several consecutive doses, you'll be at substantial risk for developing DKA.

- ✔ **You aren't taking high enough doses of insulin:** It's quite possible that day to day you give yourself a fairly similar quantity of insulin and get along quite nicely, thank you very much. That's great. But if you're experiencing some additional stress (emotional or, more commonly, physical) on your body, you will likely require higher doses of insulin to meet your body's increased needs. Examples would be if you develop, say, pneumonia or a kidney infection.

If you have type 1 diabetes, you depend on insulin injections not only to preserve your health, but to preserve your life. Even if you're feeling rotten and aren't eating anything, you *cannot* forgo taking your insulin. In fact, you may need to give yourself *more* insulin than usual. The sickest patients that diabetes specialists ever see are those people with diabetes who, unfortunately, either weren't given this advice or knew it but didn't follow it. If you have type 1 diabetes, please follow this advice. It may save your life.

Treating ketoacidosis

Ketoacidosis is a serious condition that requires very careful treatment. If you have *very mild* DKA, and you are fortunate enough to have a diabetes educator who is empowered to do this, you will possibly be treated as an outpatient under his or her very, very close supervision. The following will probably be part of your treatment:

- ✔ **Ensuring proper hydration:** Achieved by making sure you're drinking sufficient quantities of fluids.

- ✔ **Giving yourself frequent insulin injections:** You may be asked to give yourself injections of rapid-acting insulin as often as every two hours.

- ✔ **Testing your blood:** You will need to check your blood glucose and blood ketone levels often.

If you have anything more than very mild DKA, you should be treated in a hospital. The treatment will consist of the following:

- ✔ **Administering insulin:** This is usually done intravenously.

- ✔ **Ensuring proper hydration:** Achieved by intravenous administration of fluids.

- ✔ **Restoring proper potassium and mineral balance:** This is achieved by intravenous or oral administration of potassium and, at times, calcium, phosphate, magnesium, and bicarbonate.

- ✔ **Testing your blood:** Oh yes, where would we be without blood testing? You will likely be poked and prodded quite a bit, but fortunately that can usually be done by inserting a small tube into a blood vessel that can, in a sense, be turned on and off at will (sort of like a tap), so you may not have to be jabbed afresh each time.

- ✔ **Looking for the cause:** If the reason for your having developed DKA is not apparent (like missing insulin doses, for example), you may require additional blood and urine tests, X-rays, and so on to try to determine what may have triggered the episode (pneumonia, for example).

Preventing ketoacidosis

How truly wonderful it is that what was once both unavoidable (and fatal!) is now almost always avoidable. It does, however, take a fair bit of effort to accomplish this. The key measures to prevent DKA are

- **Monitor, monitor, monitor:** Often the earliest signs of developing DKA are rising blood glucose readings. If you're testing your blood frequently, you may well detect a problem before it gets out of hand.

- **Take your insulin:** Whatever you do, don't fall into the trap of figuring that if you're feeling unwell and aren't eating or drinking properly, you don't need insulin. Trust us; you *do* require insulin (possibly more than usual).

ANECDOTE

Not just cabin fever

Beth was a 13-year-old girl who had had type 1 diabetes for three years. After visiting a friend at a cottage, she came down with terrible diarrhea. She spent the better part of the day on the toilet, but with her mom's encouragement, she was able to drink lots of fluids. Beth usually required three injections of insulin per day and her total daily dose of insulin was generally about 20 units. When she became ill, her blood glucose level rose to 22 mmol/L and her blood started to test slightly positive for ketones.

Beth contacted her diabetes educator, who advised her to test her blood glucose every 2 hours and told her to take extra rapid-acting insulin every 2 hours if her blood glucose level was elevated. Over the next 12 hours she ended up taking an extra 30 units. By the next day, Beth was feeling back to normal, her glucose levels were normal, she had no ketones in the blood, her insulin doses were back to usual, and she was out playing with her friends.

Beth was thrilled. Her mom was thrilled. Her educator and her doctors were thrilled. Everyone was thrilled, in fact, except for Beth's friend, who felt terribly guilty when they found out their lake water was contaminated with giardiasis and as a result Beth had developed "beaver fever."

Hyperosmolar Hyperglycemic State

The name *hyperosmolar hyperglycemic state* refers to a situation where tremendously excessive levels of glucose are in the blood. *Hyper* means "larger than normal," *osmolar* has to do with concentrations of substances in the blood, and *glycemic* has to do with blood glucose. In other words, the blood is simply too concentrated with glucose.

Hyperosmolar hyperglycemic state (fortunately, abbreviated as HHS) occurs in people with type 2 diabetes. Like ketoacidosis, HHS is a medical emergency; unlike ketoacidosis, HHS *always* requires treatment in a hospital. (As we discuss later in this section, HHS is virtually always triggered by a serious illness — such as pneumonia, for example. Because both HHS and the illness triggering it are serious conditions, people so affected are typically very, very ill; hence the need for hospitalization.)

Hyperosmolar hyperglycemic state goes by a variety of other names, including hyperosmolar hyperglycemic nonketotic coma, hyperglycemic hyperosmolar nonketotic coma, and hyperglycemic hyperosmolar nonketotic state. What all these terms share in common is that they are a mouthful to say and impossible to remember!

Identifying the symptoms of the hyperosmolar hyperglycemic state

The symptoms of HHS arise in part from the effects on the body of very high glucose levels and in part from whatever condition (for example, a heart attack) triggered it. In terms of the high glucose levels — values as high as 100 are not unheard of — symptoms may include the following:

- ✔ Frequent urination
- ✔ Excessive thirst

✔ Dry mouth

✔ Leg cramps

✔ Weakness and lethargy

✔ Unconsciousness

The diagnosis of HHS is actually quite straightforward. If a person with known type 2 diabetes develops extraordinarily elevated blood glucose levels with evidence of dehydration and without the typical blood chemistry picture of ketoacidosis, the diagnosis is readily made.

 If you measure your blood glucose regularly — and more frequently if you are feeling unwell — you will probably never develop HHS because you'll notice if your blood glucose is getting high and you'll take corrective action before it reaches a critical level.

 HHS requires immediate and skilled treatment at a hospital. If you think you may have it, go to the nearest emergency department. The great majority of the time, however, it is not the affected person who recognizes the problem; it is a loved one (or, in the case of nursing home residents, a nurse) who detects something is wrong. The affected person is usually too sick to even know that they are unwell.

Not all elevations of blood glucose indicate HHS. If you're feeling well, you don't have the symptoms described above, and your blood glucose level is only mildly to moderately elevated (10 to 25 mmol/L or so), you probably don't have HHS. It may mean, however, that you need to speak to your health care team about improving your overall glucose control.

Examining the causes of the hyperosmolar hyperglycemic state

HHS is most common among elderly people with diabetes, though it can occur in younger individuals. Whereas ketoacidosis (see the preceding section) most often occurs when people haven't been taking sufficient insulin, HHS is most likely to occur if you have some additional serious illness that has triggered it. This illness may be, for example, a stroke, a heart attack, or a severe infection such as pneumonia.

Typically, HHS develops in an infirm person whose diabetes is reasonably well controlled until some additional factor (like those just mentioned) develops. Whereas an otherwise healthy person with type 2 diabetes would recognize the presence of the additional problem and seek medical attention, an infirm individual may not know something is amiss or may not be able to deal with it. The person then becomes increasingly unwell from the additional illness, the worsening blood glucose levels, and dehydration. Indeed, HHS leads to profound dehydration.

Treating the hyperosmolar hyperglycemic state

Similar to the treatment of ketoacidosis, HHS treatment includes the following:

- ✔ **Administering insulin:** This is usually done intravenously. (Incidentally, insulin is less important than restoring proper hydration, and often insulin can be stopped altogether within a few days.)

- ✔ **Ensuring proper hydration:** Achieved by intravenous administration of fluids. This is absolutely essential. Dehydration in HHS is usually very, very severe.

- ✔ **Restoring proper potassium and mineral balance:** This is achieved by intravenous or oral administration of potassium and, at times, calcium, phosphate, magnesium, and bicarbonate.

- ✔ **Testing your blood:** Monitoring of blood glucose levels as well as electrolytes, calcium, magnesium, phosphate, and other key blood constituents is crucial.

- ✔ **Looking for the cause:** HHS is almost always caused by something in addition to diabetes. A physician must make a meticulous search for this other cause; this search will likely include blood and urine tests, X-rays, and heart tests, among other things.

Even with the best possible therapy, the death rate for HHS is high because most people who suffer from it are elderly and have other serious illnesses that both trigger it and complicate treatment.

Preventing the hyperosmolar hyperglycemic state

Hyperosmolar hyperglycemic state can be prevented in two broad ways, depending on where you or your loved one lives:

✔ **In the community:** If you or a loved one has type 2 diabetes and lives in the community, follow the treatment plan detailed in this book. With proper therapy (including nutrition, exercise, medicines, and so forth), you will likely never develop HHS. And, importantly, if despite following proper therapy, your blood glucose levels keep climbing, contact your health care team to see if your treatment program needs to be adjusted or if a new health issue has come up that has made things worse.

✔ **In nursing homes:** If you or your loved one has diabetes and resides in a nursing home, speak to the staff (or the physician) to ensure that blood glucose levels are being checked regularly and even more often when you or your loved one is not feeling well. That way, if the blood glucose level is progressively climbing, it can be picked up rapidly and dealt with before it spirals out of control.

Chapter 2

Monitoring and Understanding Your Blood Glucose Levels

. . . .

In This Chapter

▶ Understanding the whys and wherefores of blood glucose monitoring

▶ Knowing how to use a blood glucose meter

▶ Choosing a blood glucose meter

▶ Recording your blood glucose results

▶ Knowing your blood glucose targets

▶ Interpreting your blood glucose results

▶ Assessing longer-term control with an A1C

▶ Looking at continuous glucose monitoring

. . . .

*M*any diabetes complications — such as blindness and kidney failure — are directly influenced by your blood glucose control. The better your blood glucose levels, the more likely you are to maintain your eyesight and avoid kidney failure.

But how will you know if your blood glucose levels are good? Ah, we're so glad you asked. Because that is exactly what we look at in this chapter.

Understanding the Importance of Measuring Your Blood Glucose Levels

Have you ever gotten dressed in the dark only to find out as you were heading out the door that your socks were mismatched or the blue pants you put on were actually black or your red purse was actually brown? You probably either made a mad dash back inside to re-dress, or you just headed out, hoping that your gaffe wouldn't be noticed. Well, not monitoring your blood glucose levels is like getting dressed in the dark every day.

If you are not testing your blood, you will never know if your

- ✔ Nutrition (diet) plan is helping your blood glucose control

- ✔ Exercise program is improving your blood glucose levels

- ✔ Oral hypoglycemic agents or insulin doses (see Chapter 3) need to be changed

- ✔ Recent illness, such as a chest infection, is making your glucose readings dangerously high

Basically, you'll be in the dark, without guidance and, equally important, without feedback.

But what if your readings are poor? "Why do I want to be frustrated by always seeing crummy readings?" you might ask. And you would be perfectly justified in asking this. At least, you would be perfectly justified if you couldn't improve your blood glucose control. But you can *always* improve it. If your readings aren't good, it is time for you to meet with your diabetes educators to see if your lifestyle plan needs adjusting. And it is time to call your family doctor (or diabetes specialist if you're in regular contact with one) to have your oral hypoglycemic agents or insulin therapy reviewed.

People with diabetes tend to look at a record of their glucose readings as a report card, keeping constant score and noting whether they have passed or failed. That is understandable, but terribly inappropriate. Your glucose readings aren't meant to judge you or your efforts. Your readings are being done to serve as an aid — a tool — to help you and your team know when changes to your therapy are in order. And if your readings are good, they serve as a nice source of positive feedback.

Testing your blood, not you

Ian recalls his very first meeting with Bill, a 25-year-old man who had had type 1 diabetes for several years. When Ian asked Bill how his blood glucose readings were doing, Bill told him they were excellent and pulled out his blood glucose log-book (we discuss logbooks later in this chapter) which showed his past two months' readings — all of which were within target — consistently and neatly noted. "That's great," Ian said, "why don't I borrow your blood glucose meter for a moment so that we can download your values to keep a computerized record of them in the chart?"

"Ah," Bill replied, hesitantly, "actually, I don't have my meter with me today."

"No problem," Ian replied, "maybe you could drop it off tomorrow."

"Don't think so," Bill went on, "I lost it months ago."

Bill expected recrimination, but got none. Instead, both Bill and Ian shared a knowing smile. Like having homework conveniently chewed by the household dog, people "losing" their blood glucose meter is very common. It's also common for people to make up blood glucose numbers. The reason? Because many people with diabetes have never been sufficiently taught that measuring and recording blood glucose levels are a guide — not a report card or, worse, a disciplinarian's rod. Similarly, many people with diabetes have never been sufficiently taught that their diabetes educators and doctors are more akin to guidance counsellors than truant officers. Ian made sure Bill knew this, and from then on, like Little Bo Peep, when Bill came to his appointments, his blood glucose meter and logbook were sure to follow.

Testing with a Blood Glucose Meter

You can know if your blood glucose control is where it should be through several different ways:

- ✔ Testing your blood glucose using your own portable blood glucose meter.

- ✔ Having a blood glucose test performed at a laboratory.

- ✔ Having your A1C tested at a laboratory (or, if they have an A1C testing machine, at a diabetes education centre). (See "Testing for Longer-Term Blood Glucose Control with the A1C Test," later in this chapter, for more.)

- ✔ Having your *fructosamine* level performed at a laboratory. This is a seldom-required test that indicates what your average blood glucose level has been over the preceding two weeks.

- ✔ Using a continuous glucose monitoring system (CGMS). (See "Using a Continuous Glucose Monitoring System," later in this chapter, for more.)

Of the various ways of determining your blood glucose control, far and away the easiest, most convenient method is for you to use a blood glucose meter. In this section we look in detail at how blood glucose testing with a blood glucose meter can help you manage your diabetes. (*Urine* glucose testing, by the way, is of no value in monitoring your glucose control.)

Reviewing the supplies you need

Just like any test, a blood glucose test requires some basic supplies:

- ✔ **Lancet:** If you happen to be like us, the notion of intentionally wounding yourself is most definitely not your idea of a good time. Well, you need not despair because obtaining a blood sample is a nearly painless procedure. In order to prick yourself you use a small, sharp, disposable *lancet.*

✔ **Lancet holder:** Your lancet fits into this spring-loaded holder, and when you push the release button, the lancet springs out and pokes your finger. Lancet holders are typically adjustable so that you can vary the depth the lancet will penetrate your skin. That way you can set it to the minimum depth necessary to get blood (and minimize discomfort).

✔ **Test strip:** This is the small disposable strip onto which you place your drop of blood.

✔ **Blood glucose meter:** This is the device that determines how much glucose is in your blood sample. We talk more about these in a moment.

✔ **"Sharps" container:** This is a small box into which you place your used lancets. You can pick up a sharps container from your drugstore. When the container is full, seal it and bring it back to the drugstore for proper disposal.

Also available is a lancing device (the ACCU-CHEK Multiclix Lancing Device — visit the Web site at www.accu-chek.ca), which contains a cylinder that holds several lancets. An advantage to this device is that you have less to fiddle with and it doesn't require disposal in a sharps container; when used up, it can be placed in the regular garbage.

Performing a blood glucose test

Here's how you obtain a blood sample and perform a blood glucose test:

1. **Wash your hands (or at least your finger).** Although you do not need to prepare your site — or your psyche — with alcohol, you need to make sure your finger (or arm if you are using an alternate-site meter, which we discuss in the next section) is clean.

2. **Obtain a blood sample.** Insert a lancet into the lancet holder, press it against the *side* of your fingertip, and activate the trigger. In an instant, you will see a tiny drop of blood appear. It does not hurt much at all, but to make it hurt even less you can

   • Use a lancet holder that allows you to adjust the depth of penetration.

- Avoid re-using your lancets because they dull quickly. (It's okay to use the same one a few times, but not more than that.)

    - Use the side — not the fleshy pad — of the end of your finger, and change fingers often.

    - Take blood from an alternate site such as your forearm. (To do this you will need an alternate-site meter.)

3. **Apply the end of the glucose-measuring strip to the blood.** Only a tiny drop of blood is required, but it still has to be sufficient to cover the marked area on the strip. Most strips are designed to draw up the blood in the same way that a strip of paper towel, when dipped into water, draws up the water (a process called *capillary action,* in case you were wondering).

4. **Presto, you're done!** Your meter will display your result in a matter of seconds.

If you have difficulty obtaining a sufficient quantity of blood, try one or more of the following:

- ✔ Warm your finger with warm water.

- ✔ Let your arm hang down at your side for a minute before you test.

- ✔ Hold your finger about 1.5 centimetres (about half an inch) from the tip and squeeze — but only once, as repeated squeezing can interfere with the test's accuracy.

How a blood glucose meter works

Earlier glucose meters relied on a colour change that appeared on the test strips and that was proportional to your blood glucose level. The new meters use a different process to analyze your blood. They measure an electrical potential that is created when the glucose in your blood sample reacts with reagents (glucose oxidase and potassium ferricyanide) on the electrode of the test strip. This reaction generates electrons that produce an electrical current. The higher your glucose level, the greater the current.

Because blood glucose test strips can be damaged (and thus, provide inaccurate results) if exposed to the elements, be sure to look after your unused strips as per the instructions the manufacturer provided. In particular, keep them stored in the airtight container that they came in.

If ever you find that your test result is far lower than you expect, it may be because you had insufficient blood on the strip (this can give falsely low readings). If your blood glucose meter tells you that your reading is, for example, 2.8 mmol/L and you had expected 12.8 mmol/L, retest yourself.

Incidentally, when it comes to used lancets or lancet holders (these can be contaminated with blood), remember the old adage: Neither a borrower nor a lender be. The only time you should share your blood is when you are donating to Canadian Blood Services (which, incidentally, we discuss further in Chapter 3).

Knowing how often to test your blood glucose

How often you test is determined by three factors: the kind of diabetes you have, the kind of treatment you are using, and the level of stability of your blood glucose. As you can tell, this is not a one-size-fits-all issue. The Canadian Diabetes Association (CDA) recommends different amounts of testing depending on what therapy you're taking to control your blood glucose (we share our take on this following this list):

- ✔ **If you aren't on medications to control your blood glucose (that is, you're being treated with lifestyle measures alone):** The frequency of testing should be determined (in discussion with you, your diabetes educators, and your physicians) based on your specific situation. Tests should include both before-meal and (two hours) after-meal tests.

- ✔ **If you take oral hypoglycemic agents, but not insulin:** The frequency of testing should be determined (in discussion with you, your diabetes educators, and your physicians) based on your specific situation. Tests should include both before-meal and (two hours) after-meal tests.

✔ **If you take insulin, but not oral hypoglycemic agents:** Test at least three times daily. Tests should include both before-meal and (two hours) after-meal tests.

✔ **If you take insulin once per day and also take oral hypoglycemic agents:** Test at least once daily. You should test at variable times.

"Two hours after meals" means two hours after you take the first bite of your meal.

The CDA also notes that "in many situations, for all individuals with diabetes, more frequent testing should be undertaken" because this will provide needed information to allow you and your health care team to adjust your treatment to best control your blood glucose.

The CDA recommendations are based, as they should be, on the existing science (or as Joe Friday would say, "the facts ma'am, just the facts"). However, the existing science — especially when it comes to how often testing should be done if you are not taking insulin — is pretty darn shabby. Which means, in the absence of definitive data, that patients and health care providers need to use their collective judgment in deciding how often testing is necessary. In our experience, the more you test, the more information and feedback you have, and, ultimately, the better you do. For this reason we would encourage you to focus on the "at least" wording of the CDA guidelines and aim to test considerably more often than the minimum recommendations.

We have found the following schedule to work very well (note that this schedule assumes your overall control is both very good and very stable; if it isn't, you should be testing *even more*):

✔ **If your treatment consists of lifestyle measures alone,** test *once* daily, varying the timing of your reading so that over the span of a week or two you'll have values from before and after each of your meals and at bedtime. (If your readings are uniformly within target, testing only two or three times weekly may be suitable.)

✔ **If you're taking oral hypoglycemic agents or are an adult taking insulin once or twice daily** (see Chapter 3), test *twice* daily:

- Before breakfast, *and*

- Vary the time of the other test (sometimes do it before your other meals, sometimes two hours after your meals, and sometimes at bedtime).

✔ **If you are an adult taking insulin three or four times a day (or a child or adolescent taking insulin any number of times a day),** test *four to seven* times daily:

- Before each meal, *and*

- Two hours after some meals (rotate so that one day you test after breakfast, the next day after lunch, and the next day after dinner), *and*

- *Every* night at bedtime, *and*

- *Occasionally at about 3 a.m.* (to make sure you aren't having low overnight readings that haven't been awakening you).

✔ **If you have *gestational diabetes*** (diabetes that develops during pregnancy and goes away after pregnancy ends), test before and two hours after your breakfast, two hours after your lunch, and two hours after your dinner.

✔ **If you are pregnant and have pre-existing diabetes ("pregestational diabetes"),** test *six to seven* times per day (before and two hours after each meal, and again at bedtime if your bedtime is four or more hours after your dinner, and periodically overnight).

Never fall into the trap of assuming that if you feel well, your blood glucose levels *must* be good and therefore you don't need to test. The truth is, your blood glucose level can be significantly higher than normal and you may not have a single symptom, even though your body is being irreversibly damaged.

As you can tell from this list, the frequency of testing is directly related to how often you need the information to make decisions about your care. If you're being treated with lifestyle measures alone, getting feedback once per day is usually enough to let you know how effective your treatment plan is, whereas if you're on an intensified insulin program (see Chapter 3), you should test much more often to know what insulin dose to administer.

Almost everyone has times when they get fed up with testing, testing, testing. Don't feel guilty if you feel this way; it's perfectly normal. And if you do happen to go through times when you aren't testing nearly as much as you should, don't berate yourself about it. Just grab hold of your meter and get back into the routine.

Mr. Pereira was a middle-aged man with type 2 diabetes who had come to Ian's office for a consultation. Ian asked him how his blood glucose control was, and Mr. Pereira replied, "It was 7.4 today." Ian asked him if he had any other readings to share. "Sure; it was 9.3 last month so it's getting better." Ian explained to his patient that glucose control varies not only month to month, but day to day and even meal to meal, so knowing two readings taken a month apart tells us virtually nothing about how control is or what trend it's following. Hearing this explanation, Mr. Pereira, a math teacher, asked if he could borrow Ian's calculator, and, a moment later, announced, "Gee, Doctor, now I get it. I've told you what my readings were for a total of 2 minutes out of the past 43,200 minutes. That's not even five one-thousandths of 1 percent of my readings. *No wonder* that doesn't tell you much." Couldn't have said it better ourselves.

Understanding what to do with your test results

If you test your blood glucose readings and don't share the results with your health care team and/or the results don't influence anything you do (such as adjusting your diet or exercise, or adjusting your insulin dose), you're likely to ask yourself, "Why am I bothering to test my blood?" Our answer would be, "We wonder the same thing!"

Testing your blood glucose levels is only of value if it results in some further action (even if this is only to reassure yourself, if your control is excellent, that it remains excellent). If you have a blood glucose meter, speak to your health care team about why you are testing and, importantly, what to do with the results. Without this information, we suspect you'll be likely either not to test very much or to abandon testing altogether. And we wouldn't blame you one bit.

Choosing a Blood Glucose Meter

So many meters are on the market that you may be confused about which one to use. One consideration that should play little or no part in your choice of a meter is the cost. With rebates, promotions, and trade-ins, you'll find almost every meter you look at to be quite inexpensive and competitively priced. Because the meters are so cheap and because the manufacturers replace them with better ones so frequently, you can get a new meter every year or two, to make sure that you have the latest and greatest device.

Another non-consideration is the accuracy of the various machines. All are accurate to a degree acceptable for managing your diabetes. Keep in mind, though, that they don't have the accuracy of laboratory equipment. (If ever you're experimenting with your machine and test your blood twice within a minute or two, you may find that your readings vary by 10 to 15 percent. This is not because your blood glucose level has changed that much in a matter of seconds; it's simply because the machines aren't perfect.) To make sure your blood glucose meter is sufficiently accurate, once a year your doctor (or diabetes educator) should have you do a finger-prick test with your meter at the same time as the lab is testing your glucose by drawing blood from your arm. Once the lab result is available, the two values should be compared. They should be within 20 percent of each other.

Although glucose meters are cheap, the test strips are anything but. Typically they are about a dollar per strip (ouch!), regardless of which meter you are using. If you shop around, however, you will find that some drugstores sell them for less than others.

 Some provinces and territories will subsidize the cost of your blood glucose strips. For more information you can contact your provincial or territorial government or the CDA (visit their Web site at www.diabetes.ca/get-involved/helping-you/advocacy/financial-coverage).

Because the machines are similar in price, accuracy, and costs for their strips, base your purchase decision on other factors:

✔ Whether you like products with bells and whistles or prefer those that are plain and simple.

✔ If your eyesight is poor, make sure the display is easily readable. If that is not sufficient, you can purchase a voice synthesizer that connects with a meter or, alternatively, a blood glucose meter with a built-in voice synthesizer such as the Oracle blood glucose meter (www.oraclediabetes.com).

✔ If you're likely to be testing in the dark, select a meter that has backlighting.

✔ You need to calibrate some meters (by entering a code into the machine) each time you open a new package of test strips. This is typically a fast and simple procedure, but if you think you might find it a hassle, obtain a meter that doesn't require this step. (These heavily promoted meters are referred to as requiring "no coding.")

✔ If you want to test from alternate sites such as your forearm, buy a meter designed to allow this.

✔ Make sure the meter is not too bulky (seldom an issue with current meters), or, conversely, too small to fit comfortably in your hand.

✔ Some strips are larger than others. If you have a hard time holding onto very small objects, choose a meter that uses larger strips.

✔ You'll have to decide how much memory you need in a machine. (However, we still far prefer a written log compared to any meter's memory. We discuss logbooks later in this chapter.)

✔ If you have type 1 diabetes, have a meter that tests for ketones. (See Chapter 1 for more on ketones.) The only such meter available in Canada is the Precision Xtra. This meter also tests for blood glucose.

✔ You may find a device that can hold multiple test strips more convenient.

✔ If you like the idea of being able to download your readings onto your computer so you can graph (and print) them, buy a meter that has this capacity. Bear in mind that you'll likely encounter an additional charge for the connecting cable.

The Canadian Diabetes Association offers a Consumer's Guide to Diabetes Products. This excellent publication, updated annually, is available online at www.diabetes.ca/ diabetes-and-you/literature/consumer-guide.

Alternate-site glucose readings are not reliable if they're obtained when your blood glucose level is rapidly rising or falling. For this reason, don't rely on alternate-site tests if you're doing a blood glucose test within two hours of eating, and don't use an alternate site test if you suspect you are hypoglycemic.

You'll save much time, energy, and aggravation by speaking to your diabetes educator before you buy a meter. Not only can he or she show you the latest meters and point out their pros and cons, but also, more important, your educator *knows you* and will able to help you select a meter that meets your particular needs.

If you would like to do some of your own research, you can find (far from impartial) information regarding meters by going to the different manufacturers' Web sites or by calling them. Table 2-1 lists the main manufacturers in the Canadian market, their Web sites, and phone numbers.

Table 2-1	Main Meter Manufacturers	
Company	*Web Site*	*Phone Number*
Abbott Diabetes Care	www.abbottdiabetescare.ca	888-519-6890
Auto Control Medical	www.autocontrol.com	800-461-0991
Bayer Healthcare	www.bayerdiabetes.ca	800-268-1432
Lifescan Canada	www.lifescancanada.com	800-663-5521
Roche Diagnostics	www.accu-chek.ca	800-363-7949

Recording Your Results

Ian recalls going for a haircut a few years back (when he used to have to go more often) only to find his barber profoundly upset. "What's the matter?" Ian asked, to which his barber replied that he could not find his scissors. "Why not just use somebody else's?" Ian innocently asked. His barber immediately stopped his searching and looked at Ian with disbelief. "Use somebody else's? Would you use somebody else's wife?" And that just about sums up most diabetes specialists' opinions about how glucose readings should be recorded. We're very particular and we each have our own preferences.

So then, we *could* show you many different ways of recording your results, or we could just show you the best way, which, ahem, just happens to be Ian's way!

The first thing you need to do is to obtain a logbook. You can find these at your pharmacy, at your diabetes education centre, and at your diabetes specialist's office. Each page in your logbook should be laid out like Figure 2-1 (of course, if you're not on insulin you won't use the right hand side of the page).

	Blood Glucose Levels									Insulin Injections						Notes
Date	Breakfast		Lunch		Dinner		Bedtime	Other	Insulin Type	Units Taken						
	Before	After	Before	After	Before	After				Breakfast	Lunch	Dinner	Bedtime			

Figure 2-1: Ideal logbook format.

Most logbooks, alas, do not have this particular format. If you can't find a book with this layout, you can download similar pages from Ian's Web site (www.ourdiabetes.com/log-book.htm).

The one shortcoming with this layout is, potentially, insufficient space for you to write in the Notes column (where you might want to write things such as "birthday party" or "missed snack" to remind you later of some past event that might explain a high or low reading). If you need more space, you can always create your own sheet on a piece of paper (which you could photocopy) or with a spreadsheet program such as Excel.

Using this layout enables you to quickly assess your overall blood glucose *patterns, trends,* and *averages* for a given time of day. To illustrate what we mean, have a look at two different ways of recording your readings.

Table 2-2 is the typical way that a log is kept or that a machine's memory displays results (although a machine would usually display the time of day, not the meal of the day). The readings in this table are before-meal values.

Table 2-2	Blood Glucose Readings Listed Chronologically
Time of Reading	*Blood Glucose Level*
Breakfast	12.6
Lunch	4.1
Dinner	14.7
Bedtime	5.6
Breakfast	11.7
Lunch	5.2
Dinner	12.1
Bedtime	7.0
Breakfast	10.0
Lunch	5.9
Dinner	11.9
Bedtime	4.0
Breakfast	9.9
Lunch	4.2
Dinner	14.4
Bedtime	4.4
Breakfast	11.1
Lunch	6.3
Dinner	12.2
Bedtime	5.1

If you were to record your readings like this, you would likely feel that your glucose values were all over the place (or, as Ian often hears, "my sugars are up and down like a toilet seat") and you would likely be feeling frustrated by what you concluded were very inconsistent values. Although your conclusion would be perfectly understandable, you might be surprised to see that if we look at your readings from a different perspective, they could be thought of as being remarkably consistent. Table 2-3 takes those same readings and charts them differently.

Table 2-3	Blood Glucose Reading Listed by Time of Day		
Breakfast	*Lunch*	*Dinner*	*Bedtime*
12.6	4.1	14.7	5.6
11.7	5.2	12.1	7.0
10.0	5.9	11.9	4.0
9.9	4.2	14.4	4.4
11.1	6.3	12.2	5.1

Now, scan the columns from top to bottom. Aha! Your readings at any given time of day are remarkably similar. You're consistently too high at breakfast, consistently normal at lunch, consistently too high at dinner, and consistently normal at bedtime.

The memory on a blood glucose meter does not allow for this type of instant overview, and hence is almost always inferior to using a logbook.

Record keeping is of great importance because when you have identified your blood glucose patterns, your health care team can adjust your therapy accordingly. In the preceding example, if you were on insulin therapy, we would know that you need more bedtime insulin to bring down your breakfast blood glucose and, depending on the type of insulin you are taking, more lunchtime or breakfast insulin to reduce your suppertime readings (see Chapter 3 for a detailed discussion of insulin adjustment). We could have figured this out from Table 2-2, but it would have been much more difficult and time-consuming. We discuss how to interpret blood glucose log readings in the section "Interpreting Your Blood Glucose Results," later in this chapter.

If you're using an insulin pump (see Chapter 3) you may need an even more detailed logbook; ask your diabetes educator for his or her recommended one.

Bring your logbook with you to *each and every* appointment with your diabetes educator and diabetes specialist. Ask your family doctor how often he or she would like you to bring your logbook to your appointments (if you see your doctor only occasionally, he or she will want you to bring it routinely, but on the other hand, if you're seeing him or her very frequently for other health issues — such as, for example, allergy injections — your doctor likely won't need to review your readings at each of these visits).

Discovering Your Blood Glucose Targets

The Canadian Diabetes Association (CDA) guidelines recommend that most adults with type 1 or type 2 diabetes aim for the following readings:

Before Meals	*Two Hours after Meals*
4–7 mmol/L	5–10 mmol/L

However, if your A1C is above 7.0 (we discuss A1C later in this chapter in the section "Testing for Longer-Term Blood Glucose Control with the A1C Test"), the CDA recommends aiming for a lower two-hour after-meal target of 5–8 mmol/L.

Not everyone can safely achieve these targets. Here are some of the things that might make it unsafe or inappropriate for you to aim for these levels:

- ✔ You have other health problems that make it too dangerous to risk any hypoglycemia.

- ✔ You have *irreversible* problems with hypoglycemia unawareness (see Chapter 1).

- ✔ When you try to bring your blood glucose into this range, you experience excessively *frequent, unpredictable, and unavoidable* hypoglycemia.

- ✔ Your life expectancy is such that you're at low risk of developing diabetes-related, long-term complications.

No one with diabetes has glucose readings that are always within target. Indeed, having two-thirds of your readings within target is a wonderful accomplishment. Remember that to achieve your targets requires a concerted and ongoing effort by you and your diabetes team. (And also remember, *you* are the first star on this team.)

Consistently achieving target blood glucose values can be very difficult and, for some people, it may simply not be possible. If you and your health care team have worked hard at reaching these goals but have not been able to achieve them, don't feel that all is lost. The reason for this is simple; although fantastic blood glucose readings are our goal, *any* improvement in your blood glucose control will help reduce your risk of microvascular complications (such as blindness and kidney failure) and, possibly, macrovascular complications (such as heart attack and stroke).

Interpreting Your Blood Glucose Results

In the section "Understanding the Importance of Measuring Your Blood Glucose Levels" earlier in this chapter, we mention that testing your blood glucose (and recording your results) is only of value if something is then done with the results. Otherwise, it's a waste of your time — and an expensive waste at that.

Because your diabetes educators and physicians know you and are aware of your particular circumstances (including your medications), they can provide you with advice that is specific to you. (That is, they can help you determine what your specific blood glucose targets are and how you can best go about achieving them.) Nonetheless, certain basic principles can help guide you. The most important of these is to look for patterns in your blood glucose levels, and the first step in doing this is to record your values in the format we show in Table 2-3. In this section we look at three particularly common problematic patterns you might spot in your results and how you can improve these problems.

When your before-breakfast readings are high (and other readings good)

As we discover in Chapter 3, one particularly common scenario is for people with diabetes (regardless of their treatment) to have higher readings first thing in the morning than later in the day. A typical logbook might look like Figure 2-2.

Date	Breakfast		Lunch		Dinner		Bedtime
	Bef.	After	Bef.	After	Bef.	After	
	8.5	7.2					
	9.0		6.1				
	7.8			5.2			
	6.1				4.4		
	8.2					7.9	
	9.9						8.2

Figure 2-2: High before-breakfast (fasting) blood glucose readings.

The reason for this pattern is that overnight your liver produces and releases glucose into your blood (this is called the *dawn phenomenon*). Often, the best way to treat this increased before-breakfast glucose level is by taking a dose of insulin (NPH, Levemir, or Lantus) before you go to bed (sometimes these insulins are given at other times instead) or, if you are already taking one of these insulins, by increasing the dose (under the guidance of your diabetes educator or physician).

When your after-meal readings are high (and other readings good)

You may observe that your readings are good before your meals but two hours after your meals your values have climbed. Your logbook might look something like Figure 2-3.

Date	Breakfast		Lunch		Dinner		Bedtime
	Bef.	After	Bef.	After	Bef.	After	
	5.5	8.2					
	6.0		6.1				
	7.0			8.8			
	6.1				4.4		
	4.2					9.9	
	5.9						7.2

Figure 2-3: High two-hour after-meal blood glucose readings.

In this case, the first thing to do is to review your diet with your dietitian, because your choice of foods may be responsible. Alternatively, if you're taking oral hypoglycemic agents, you might benefit from using one (such as GlucoNorm) that specifically targets after-meal blood glucose spikes. Another very effective measure is to take rapid-acting insulin (Apidra, Humalog, or NovoRapid) before your meals. If you're having this blood glucose problem despite already taking one of these medicines, then your dose(s) may need to be adjusted. (We discuss insulin adjustment in greater detail in Chapter 3.)

When your readings have no pattern

Perhaps your blood glucose readings are inconsistent, and really have no discernable pattern at all. High then low, up then down; resembling (and making you feel like you're on) a roller coaster. Your logbook may look something like Figure 2-4.

Date	Breakfast		Lunch		Dinner		Bedtime	Other
	Bef.	After	Bef.	After	Bef.	After		
	4.1	8.2						3.5
	12.5		4.2			19.9		7.7
	3.2			14.7				
	16.5				24.4		5.4	
	6.7		13.4			9.9		
	11.2			2.6			7.2	

Figure 2-4: Inconsistent blood glucose readings.

Fortunately, some correctable or at least modifiable factor is almost always present that, when addressed, can improve this situation.

If you're having wide and unpredictable swings in your glucose levels, get in touch with your diabetes specialist and your diabetes educators. They will be able to help sort out the reasons for the problem. It is rare indeed that erratic glucose control cannot be improved.

These are possible causes of erratic blood glucose levels:

✔ **Your nutrition plan isn't optimal for you.** If your nutrition program isn't working out the way it should, it's time for another visit to the dietitian. It could be that your food selection or amount might need to be changed, or it could be that you would benefit from carbohydrate counting (see Chapter 3) or using lower glycemic index foods.

✔ **Your adherence to your nutrition plan needs some work.** Are you eating *in*consistently? Do you eat almost nothing all day and then consume the bulk of your calories at suppertime? Do you graze from the time you get home in the evening until you go to bed? All these patterns can adversely affect glucose control. Also, eating disorders are not uncommon for teenage girls and young women with diabetes and can wreck havoc on blood glucose control.

✔ **Your exercise pattern needs to be revised.** Are you exercising for 10 minutes one morning and then 30 minutes the next evening and then 15 minutes the next afternoon and then not at all for two days? Consistent duration and timing of exercise is often helpful in maintaining consistent glucose control.

✔ **You have diabetic gastroparesis or celiac disease.** These conditions cause erratic absorption of nutrients into the body, and as a result can cause overly variable blood glucose readings.

✔ **You are under undue stress.** Stress does not cause diabetes, but it can certainly influence it. Stress causes the release of certain hormones in your body, including cortisol and adrenaline, both of which can make glucose levels rise. If you're on an emotional roller coaster, your glucose readings may be too.

✔ **Your menstrual cycle.** For some women with diabetes, where they are in their cycle can influence their glucose control. Some women find their glucose readings are higher around the time of their period and some find their readings are lower. Most women don't find much difference.

✔ **Your work schedule.** If you work a variable shift, you may find your readings are also variable. As most people with diabetes quickly find out, diabetes loves consistency. Nonetheless, working variable shifts does not make excellent glucose control impossible, just more difficult. If you work variable shifts, we recommend basal-bolus or pump therapy (see Chapter 3).

Another very important reason for inconsistent blood readings, as seen in Figure 2-4, is that your insulin therapy isn't working sufficiently well for you. You may need to

✔ **Change to a different type of insulin or a different insulin regimen.** Different insulins have different properties and, like the expression, "different strokes for different folks," you need to take the insulin that most closely matches your needs and works best for you. For example:

  • If you're taking NPH insulin and have inconsistent blood glucose readings, switching to Lantus or Levemir may be helpful because both are absorbed more consistently than NPH and as a result can give more consistent blood glucose control.

- If you have type 1 diabetes but are only on twice-daily insulin, your blood glucose control is almost guaranteed to be erratic, and switching to basal-bolus therapy (this is closer to normal insulin release from the pancreas; see Chapter 3) is recommended. (This is also often helpful if you have type 2 diabetes.)

- If you're having erratic readings despite basal-bolus injection therapy, switching to insulin pump therapy may provide you with much more consistent blood glucose control.

✔ **Not miss insulin doses.** If you're missing insulin doses due to forgetfulness, set reminders for yourself when your insulin is due or ask others to remind you. If you are omitting insulin doses by intention (as is not uncommonly done by teenage girls to help them lose weight), this is very, very dangerous and must not be done. If this applies to you, speak to your diabetes educator or physician urgently to see what other, safer measures can help you keep your weight in check.

✔ **Better mix your insulin.** Cloudy insulins such as NPH need to be properly mixed before you inject them (see Chapter 3).

✔ **Make sure your insulin hasn't lost its potency.** If your insulin has been exposed to excessive cold or heat, or is beyond its expiry date, it will have lost its potency and should not be used.

✔ **Change the place you are injecting your insulin because of problems with insulin absorption.** You may give yourself the same dose of insulin every day (something, by the way, that's seldom a good idea, as we discuss earlier in this chapter), but that doesn't mean that your bloodstream sees the same dose. Factors that can affect the rate of absorption of insulin from your injection sites include the following:

  - Whether your injection sites have scar tissue. You shouldn't inject insulin into these areas.

  - Whether your injection sites have fat build-up (*lipohypertrophy*). Insulin absorption will vary considerably injection-to-injection if given into these areas. Also, injecting into them makes the lipohypertrophy worse. You shouldn't inject insulin into these areas.

- Which part of your body you are injecting into (regular insulin will begin to work more quickly if injected into the abdomen than into the arms or legs). Speak to your diabetes educator about the best locations to inject your insulin and how often you should change the sites you use.

- Whether you exercise a certain part of your body after you inject there. If, for example, you inject regular insulin into your leg and then go for a run, the rate of insulin absorption will speed up. It's best not to inject insulin into a limb that is about to be exercised.

- Whether you're accidentally injecting into muscle. (This would cause the insulin to be absorbed faster.)

The list of possible causes of overly variable blood glucose readings is lengthy indeed. One term, however, that is missing from the list is *brittle diabetes.* We consider this, in general, to be a four letter word. *Brittle diabetes* can be defined as erratic and disabling blood glucose variability occurring for no known reason and defying improvement. Although we often are referred patients with erratic blood glucose readings (some of whom have been labelled as having brittle diabetes), there is *almost always a cause* and *almost always a way to make it better.* For a doctor (or other health care provider or, indeed, for a person with diabetes) to simply attribute erratic blood glucose control to brittle diabetes without first carefully looking for (and treating) any and all possible causes such as those in the preceding list is, in our opinion, not only a shame, but a travesty. (Not that we feel strongly about this or anything.)

Testing for Longer-Term Blood Glucose Control with the A1C Test

Individual blood glucose tests are great for telling you how you're doing at a specific moment in time, but they don't give you the big picture. Frequent blood glucose measurements help, but even then, they only provide a series of snapshots of your glucose levels. So what you need is a test that gives an estimate of your *overall* control over a longer period of time. And that's precisely what can be determined from a test called an A1C. Your *A1C* is a measure of how much glucose has become attached to your red blood cells over approximately the preceding three (to four) months.

Knowing your A1C is crucial because the likelihood of your developing microvascular complications (that is, eye, kidney, and nerve damage) is directly related to your A1C. A normal A1C reading is 6 or less. An A1C of 7 or less is very good and puts you at quite low risk for microvascular damage. An A1C of 9 or higher is poor and puts you at much greater risk. An A1C that is too high is an alarm to you and your health care team that you need to improve your control. If you can drop your A1C by even 1 percent, you'll substantially decrease your risk of microvascular complications. One landmark study found that reducing the A1C by just 1 percent (equivalent to a reduction in average blood glucose of only 2 mmol/L) resulted in an astounding 37 percent lower risk of microvascular complications.

You may come across other terms for A1C, including *hemoglobin A1C, glycosylated hemoglobin,* or *glycohemoglobin.* You may also come across it abbreviated as HbA1C or HgbA1C. These all mean the same thing. Also you may find an A1C written as a number (9, for example) or as a percentage (9 %, for example); both of these are correct and mean the same thing.

After you have had your A1C tested, be sure you contact your doctor (or diabetes educator, if he or she is the one who requested the test) to find out the result. If your A1C is above target (we discuss targets later in this section), be sure to ask your diabetes educator, diabetes specialist, and/or family physician what steps you can take to improve your result.

The A1C test doesn't replace blood glucose meter testing; it's *complementary* to it. Because the A1C represents an overall estimate of your blood glucose control, it doesn't express how many highs and lows you may be having. Your average glucose level may be good even though half your readings are too low and the other half too high. It's sort of like having one foot in ice water and the other in boiling water and saying, "On average, I feel fine."

Table 2-4 shows what the average blood glucose levels are (over the preceding three to four months) for a given A1C.

Table 2-4	A1C with Corresponding Average Blood Glucose Level
A1C	*Average Blood Glucose (in mmol/L)*
5	5.4
6	7.0
7	8.6
8	10.2
9	11.8
10	13.4
11	14.9
12	16.5

TECHNICAL STUFF

How A1C works

Within red blood cells is a protein called *hemoglobin*. Hemoglobin carries oxygen around the body, delivering it to where it is needed to assist with various chemical reactions that are taking place. Hemoglobin is constantly exposed to the glucose within the blood and becomes permanently attached to it. It attaches in several different ways, and the total of all the hemoglobin attached to glucose is called *glyco-hemoglobin*. The largest fraction, two-thirds of the glycohemoglobin, is in a form called hemoglobin A1C. This is the easiest form to measure.

The rest of the hemoglobin is made up of hemoglobins A1a and A1b. The more glucose in the blood, the more glycohemoglobin forms.

Hemoglobin is destroyed when the red blood cell that contains it dies. This occurs after the red blood cell has been in existence for about 120 days or so. Because glycohemo-globin remains in the blood for that length of time, it is a reflection of the glucose control over that entire time period and not just the second that a single glucose test reflects.

As the table demonstrates, the higher your A1C, the higher your blood glucose levels have been running. The lower your A1C, the lower your recent blood glucose levels.

As you can see, your A1C reading is not the same as your average blood glucose reading. This is commonly misunderstood. (For example, an A1C of 8.0 does *not* mean that your average blood glucose level is 8.0 mmol/L; it actually corresponds to average readings of 10.2 mmol/L.) (To help alleviate this confusion, a new way of looking at average blood glucose is on the horizon: the estimated average glucose. To learn more about this new measurement, have a look at the sidebar "Estimated average glucose.")

The Canadian Diabetes Association recommends that most adults with diabetes have their A1C tested every three months; the target A1C for most adults with diabetes is 7 or less. (If you are pregnant it will need to be checked more often, and your goal is lower.)

As long as you use your blood glucose meter frequently, your A1C result will likely be as anticipated. When it isn't (for example, if your meter's average was 7.0 mmol/L yet your A1C was 10), you and your health care team will need to figure out why. The most common reason for this is that your readings are up when you aren't testing and therefore you wouldn't be aware of the elevations. If your readings have this sort of discrepancy, try testing more often and at times you haven't been testing (including overnight). On occasion, an A1C is affected by other substances in the blood or by anemia. If your physician suspects this, he or she can contact the laboratory to discuss this possibility.

Apart from going to the lab to have them take blood from your arm, you can check your A1C in two other ways. Some diabetes centres have a desktop machine that can process a finger-prick sample in six minutes so that you (and they) will know your result while you are there for your visit. The cost is usually about $10 per test.

Estimated average glucose

As of August 2008, the American Diabetes Association has adopted a new way of looking at average blood glucose control, called *estimated average glucose (eAG)*. We expect that over the next few years this term will become increasingly adopted and the term A1C will become less and less often used (except in scientific discussions).

In the future you will no longer be told, for example, that your A1C is, say, 7.0. Instead you will be told — in

this particular example — that your estimated average glucose is 8.6. Estimated average glucose, as the name suggests, is the estimate of your average blood glucose for approximately the preceding three months. It's a value derived from the A1C using a simple formula. You can find both the formula and, even better, an online A1C-to-eAG calculator at http://professional.diabetes.org/glucosecalculator.aspx.

Using a Continuous Glucose Monitoring System

One of the neatest things to come along over the past few years in the world of diabetes management is continuous glucose monitoring (CGM), performed using a continuous glucose monitoring system (CGMS). We expect this technology will, sometime in the not-too-distant future, revolutionize the way that diabetes management is performed, initially for people using insulin pump therapy and, ultimately, for most people with diabetes.

Continuous glucose monitoring is, as its name suggests, the continuous measuring of your glucose level. Because it is continuous it is also referred to as real-time glucose monitoring. We discuss the different aspects of CGM in this section.

Understanding continuous glucose monitoring

A CGMS consists of three components: a sensor, a transmitter, and a receiver (or display; see Figure 2-5). The currently available CGMS in Canada has two types of receiver: One that is solely dedicated to this role, or one that is integrated into an insulin pump.

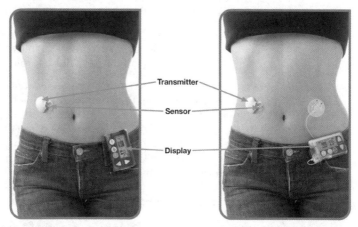

Figure 2-5: Guardian REAL-Time Continuous Glucose Monitoring System.

Here's how the different components of a CGMS work:

✓ **Sensor:** A sensor is a disposable device with an electrode-containing tiny tail that's inserted under the skin — typically on the abdomen or buttock, but you can also put it on your arm or leg. Like your blood glucose test strips, the sensor measures your glucose level; however, unlike your blood glucose test strips, it measures your glucose level in your *interstitial* fluid, not your blood. The sensor then passes this information along to the transmitter.

✔ **Transmitter:** The sensor is directly connected to the transmitter. The transmitter receives your glucose level reading from the sensor and, using radio frequency technology, sends this data to the display (receiver).

✔ **Receiver (Display):** The display, well, displays. It shows your current glucose level, your glucose levels over the past number of hours, and whether your glucose level is going up or down (this is indicated by arrows pointing — as you might imagine — up or down), and it also has an alarm that will alert you if your glucose level is too low or too high. (The alarm thresholds are adjustable.)

The display updates every five minutes; that means you will have a total of 288 measurements displayed per 24 hours. (Imagine doing 288 finger-prick samples per day!)

Because the display is wireless, it can be kept anywhere up to several feet from the transmitter. This means that at night, for instance, you can put it on your bedside table and it'll still work. The receiver's data (your glucose levels) can also be downloaded to a computer for reviewing or uploaded to a Web site where both you and your health care team can review it.

The inside scoop on how a CGMS works

The sensor component of a CGMS doesn't, in and of itself, determine your glucose level. Rather, every ten seconds, the sensor captures, in the form of an electrical signal, raw data from the interstitial fluid (similar to the way Environment Canada weather balloons capture raw data from their measuring devices in the atmosphere). The sensor's raw data is passed to the transmitter, which, every five minutes averages the data and then sends packets of this raw data to the receiver. The receiver then takes this raw data and converts it into a glucose level result (similar to the way a TV meteorologist takes Environment Canada's raw data and interprets it and then displays it as the beautiful illustrations we see on television).

Checking out the benefits of continuous glucose monitoring

No matter how often you test your blood, you won't know what your glucose levels are for much of the day. This could mean you're not aware of significant periods of time when your glucose level is outside of the target range (we discuss target blood glucose levels earlier in this chapter). This is especially concerning if you have hypoglycemia unawareness (see Chapter 1) and, thus, don't recognize when you have low blood glucose.

A CGMS helped Martha, a patient of Ian's, who was testing her blood frequently using a blood glucose meter. (Her test results are marked as *x*'s in Figure 2-6.)

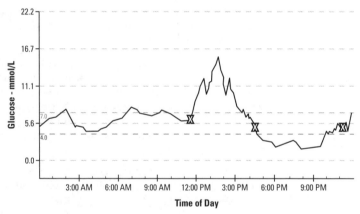

Figure 2-6: Results from a continuous glucose monitor.

Martha's blood glucose levels, measured using her blood glucose meter, were excellent and, indeed, consistently within target. Her A1C was also excellent (6.5). However the continuous line in the graph — which represents the data obtained from her CGMS — reveals that she had elevated blood glucose from about noon until 3 p.m., and low blood glucose from

7 p.m. to 10 p.m. If Martha and Ian relied exclusively on her blood glucose meter results, they would have mistakenly thought everything was fine, whereas, in fact, her levels were often high and often low. Using the information from the CGMS, Ian, Martha, and her diabetes educators were able to adjust her insulin doses and diet, and her glucose levels were much more consistent thereafter.

Here are some of the ways that CGM can help you:

- By providing you with a continuous display of your glucose levels, it gives you immediate feedback to tell you how something you eat or some exercise you do is affecting your glucose control. This will then allow you to modify your diet, your exercise, or your insulin dosing if necessary.

- Up and down trending arrows will alert you to an impending high or low blood glucose level so you can take corrective action before your glucose level gets too far out of whack.

- By having an alarm that sounds (and vibrates) if your glucose level is too low (you can adjust the alarm setting; most people set it at about 4.5 or so), you will be alerted to an impending episode of hypoglycemia before it happens. This is especially helpful for people who experience hypoglycemia during their sleep or who have hypoglycemia unawareness.

- By having an alarm that goes off if your glucose level is too high (again, you can adjust this), you will be alerted when you might need to take extra insulin.

Looking at the drawbacks of continuous glucose monitoring

Like all technology — especially new technology — CGM has some shortcomings. These include the following:

- **Cost:** Only one brand of CGMS is currently available in Canada. (Others are available in the United States.) The available sensors cost about $50. The one sensor currently available in Canada is approved by Health Canada for use for no more than three days, at which time it's supposed to be replaced. There is, however, little (if any) significant risk of using it for longer periods of time and, being the frugal souls that people are, most all CGMS users (uneventfully) use their sensors for six days or even longer. The available transmitter (which needs to be replaced every nine months or so) is about $700. The cost of the receiver/display unit is another $1,000 or so, but is much less expensive if integrated into an insulin pump (a sensor augmented pump).

✔ **Discomfort:** Some people find that inserting the sensor is uncomfortable or even somewhat painful. This is typically fleeting.

✔ **Inaccuracy:** Sensors are very accurate, but not perfectly so. Indeed, on occasion a value can be way off. For this reason, if you get a value that's low enough or high enough that you would need to take corrective action (for example, say your sensor tells you that your glucose level is 20 mmol/L), you must first do a blood glucose meter test to verify that you are truly this high before, in this example, giving yourself extra insulin. (Just imagine if the sensor told you your glucose level was 20 — and you gave extra insulin — but in reality your glucose level was only 4. This would be very dangerous.)

✔ **Time lag:** Sensors measure the glucose level in your interstitial fluid (just under the skin surface), not in your blood. Most of the time the source is not important because interstitial fluid and blood have similar glucose levels. However, when your blood glucose level is quickly rising (such as immediately after eating) or quickly falling, your interstitial glucose level is different from your blood level. (It takes about 15 minutes for the interstitial fluid glucose level to catch up to the blood glucose level.) For this reason, you may notice symptoms of hypoglycemia, for example, even though the number you see on the display is not low because the interstitial fluid glucose has yet to catch up. When you suspect your glucose level differs from what you see on the display, you'll need to test your blood to be certain what your level truly is.

✔ **Calibration:** The sensors need to be taught how to interpret interstitial glucose readings. The way you teach them is by, typically twice per day, doing a blood glucose test and entering the result into the CGMS. For this and for the other reasons detailed in this list, having a CGMS does not mean you can throw away your blood glucose meter and lancets.

Despite its shortcomings, CGM can be a life-altering and life-enhancing technology. One of Ian's patients had such severe problems with recurring severe hypoglycemia that an ambulance was visiting her house three times per week. She obtained a CGMS, and thereafter, whenever her levels were heading low, her alarm went off so that she could treat her impending hypoglycemia before it got out of hand. She didn't require a single ambulance visit once she started using the device.

CGM is far from perfect, but every year the technology improves and ultimately this will lead to the development of a feedback loop (essentially, an artificial pancreas) wherein your glucose sensor will continually and reliably measure your glucose level and automatically instruct your insulin pump to give just the right amount of insulin to match your needs. As one of Ian's patients said, "I'll simply have my pancreas outside of my body instead of inside my body."

Finding out more about CGM

You can learn more about CGM by checking out Medtronic's Web site (www.minimed.ca). Medtronic makes the Guardian REAL-Time Continuous Glucose Monitoring System and the MiniMed Paradigm REAL-Time Insulin Pump and Continuous Glucose Monitoring System, the only CGMS currently available in Canada.

Chapter 3

Using Insulin Effectively

In This Chapter

▶ Understanding how insulin works

▶ Discovering the different types of insulin

▶ Using insulin therapy for type 1 diabetes

▶ Using insulin therapy for type 2 diabetes

▶ Tackling insulin myths

▶ Figuring out how to take insulin

▶ Taking proper care of your insulin

▶ Altering your insulin dosage

▶ Dealing with erratic blood glucose readings

▶ Travelling with your insulin

*T*he discovery of insulin over 80 years ago was rightly heralded as a miraculous event. Indeed, since Banting, Best, Macleod, and Collip's famous breakthrough in 1921, the lives of tens of millions of people have been enhanced or, often, saved as a direct result of insulin therapy. However, as the years have passed, along with insulin's justified reputation as a *miracle,* so, too has insulin come for many people to be thought of as being something dangerous and scary. In this chapter we look at the many benefits insulin therapy has to offer and we clear up misconceptions surrounding one of Canada's most famous contributions to the world.

What Is Insulin?

If you're a person with type 1 diabetes, insulin is your saviour. Simply put, without insulin you could not survive. And if you have type 2 diabetes, though insulin may not very often be the difference between life and death (not in the short term, anyhow), it frequently is the difference between good health and bad health. *Insulin* is a hormone that's produced in the pancreas and released into the bloodstream, where it travels to different parts of your body. Insulin acts on certain cells (such as fat cells and muscle cells) to allow glucose to enter so that they can carry out their normal functions. If you don't have insulin in your body to allow glucose to enter into the tissues, the glucose hangs around in the blood, damages your organs, and starts to spill out into your urine.

We measure injected insulin in units. Nowadays medical science has very scientific ways of determining the strength of insulin with laboratory machinery. We've come a long way from the time that a unit of insulin was based on how much insulin it took to cause a 2-kg rabbit to have severe enough hypoglycemia that it would have a seizure.

Moving away misperceptions: How Dorothy overcame her fears about insulin

Dorothy Strait was 50 when she was diagnosed with type 2 diabetes. Her initial treatment was lifestyle therapy, and she was thrilled when a change in her diet, modest weight loss, and a daily walk brought her glucose levels down to normal. A couple of years later, however, her glucose levels started to climb and she began taking oral hypoglycemic agents. That helped, but only temporarily, and her glucose readings had now risen to 11 and she was feeling fatigued. Her family doctor referred her to Ian to see if she should be on insulin. When Dorothy came to Ian's office, she was sad, angry, and frightened all at once. She felt like a failure. She was terrified of the needle and told Ian, "I would hate jabbing myself. I simply couldn't do it. You can't convince me otherwise." As she spoke to Ian she was on the verge of tears.

"Dorothy," Ian said, "we will do whatever you want. I can't force you to do anything. And I wouldn't want to even if I could. You are the boss and you will decide what you want to do. But I think you would be unfair to yourself if, whatever you decide, it wasn't an informed decision. So let's make sure you know the most important information to help you make your decision." Dorothy was certainly agreeable to that.

Ian said a few things to Dorothy that day. He remembers telling her, "It is crucial that you know that you are not a failure, your pancreas is, and that's not your fault. It happens to most people with diabetes. And as for hating jabbing yourself, why would you like it? Who would? But you are already jabbing yourself each time you test your blood glucose.

And doing a blood finger jab is more uncomfortable than giving insulin. With the tiny needles we use nowadays, giving insulin is virtually pain free. And as for not being able to do it, look at the other obstacles that you have overcome; you've changed your diet, you've lost some weight, you're exercising regularly, you're taking a whole bunch of pills that I'm sure you'd rather not have to, and you're testing your blood every day. You've managed all those things. And if you can handle all those things, I'm sure you could manage giving insulin also."

Dorothy became more at ease but was still apprehensive. "But, Doctor, when you start insulin, you're on it forever."

"That's usually true, Dorothy," Ian replied, "but not because insulin is addictive. It's because your pancreas is failing and it's not going to be rejuvenated. It can no longer make enough insulin, so we have to supplement it. We're simply giving your body back the hormone it's lacking. One other thing: Medical science is always progressing. Other ways of giving insulin are being developed. Better pills are always coming along. I don't know if you'll be on insulin injections forever. Maybe in a few years you won't have to be."

Well, Dorothy still wasn't thrilled with the prospect of giving insulin. And of course there was no reason for her to be thrilled. But she met with the diabetes educator and was pleasantly surprised to find that giving insulin wasn't nearly as bad as she had thought. It wasn't fun by any means, but it wasn't horrible either. And as her glucose levels returned to normal and her energy improved, she was very glad she had decided to take insulin after all.

Looking at the Types of Insulin

Our pancreas normally functions on autopilot. When we eat, our blood glucose level goes up and our pancreas immediately responds by releasing insulin into the bloodstream, which promptly brings our glucose level back to normal. If your pancreas is malfunctioning and you require insulin injections, the goal is to try to reproduce what your pancreas would normally do if it was healthy. You can consider this "thinking like a pancreas." We're aided by having a variety of different insulins to choose from, each with its own set of properties. When you're prescribed insulin, your doctor should try to match your body's needs with the most appropriate insulin (or, if you have type 2 diabetes, oftentimes, the most appropriate combination of insulin and oral hypoglycemic agents). Because each person is different, the type of insulin you first start on may be changed to a different one depending on how your body responds.

The discovery of insulin

Until not too long ago, type 2 diabetes was uncommon. To have diabetes was to have type 1 diabetes. And to have type 1 diabetes before the discovery of insulin was to have a terminal illness. Imagine, therefore, the euphoria that greeted the discovery of insulin. It must surely have been equal to what the discovery of a universal cure for cancer would be nowadays. And it happened right here in Canada.

In 1889, a scientist discovered that if a dog's pancreas was removed, the dog became diabetic. This was the first strong clue that the pancreas and diabetes were intimately related. But how they were related remained a mystery.

In 1920, Dr. Frederick Banting, a Canadian surgeon from Alliston, Ontario, was working as a very junior lecturer at the University of Western Ontario in London. While preparing for a class, he read an article on diabetes and the pancreas, and that sparked an interest — soon to be an obsession — in finding out what secretion the pancreas might be making that prevents diabetes.

Dr. Banting, all of 29 years of age at the time, approached Dr. John Macleod, a professor at the University of Toronto, and asked permission to use a laboratory. Dr. Macleod agreed and assigned Charles H. Best, a science student, to assist. How was Best chosen for a role that was soon to make him world-famous? Through a rigorous selection process, you might think. Well, it wasn't quite like that. In fact, Best was picked by virtue of winning a coin toss!

Dr. Banting and Mr. Best (he wasn't a doctor yet) began their work in May 1921, and in December they were joined by J. B. Collip, a biochemist from the University of Alberta. After some initial setbacks (What would science be without setbacks?), they eventually purified a pancreatic extract that they felt could be given to people with diabetes.

On January 11, 1922, their extract was administered to Leonard Thompson, a 14-year-old boy in the Toronto General Hospital. The treatment was a dismal failure. Thankfully, the young scientists and Leonard were not deterred and, after some further work in the laboratory, they tried again on January 23. We do not know if they shouted "Eureka!" but they must have wanted to when they saw Leonard's glucose level fall and his well-being suddenly improve. The boy had been rescued from death. Insulin was born.

That is the end of one story and the beginning of another, for the subsequent personal rivalries between Banting and Best on the one side and Collip and Macleod on the other is the stuff of legend. The Nobel Prize in physiology or medicine was awarded to Banting and Macleod in 1923. Banting shared his portion with

Best, and Macleod did likewise with Collip. Michael Bliss, a Canadian historian, has written an absolutely wonderful book, *The Discovery of Insulin,* which chronicles the story and is as entertaining and fascinating to read as any detective novel you're likely to come across.

Insulins (and their properties) available in Canada are listed in Table 3-1. Note that the times given are approximations and can vary significantly — even for the same person.

Table 3-1   Types of Insulin Available in Canada and Their Properties

Classification	Generic Name	Trade Name(s)	Onset of Action	Peak Action	Duration of Action
Rapid-acting	aspart	Novorapid	10 to 15 minutes	1 to 2 hours	3 to 5 hours
	glulisine	Apidra			
	lispro	Humalog			
Short-acting	regular	Humulin-R Novolin ge Toronto	30 minutes	2 to 3 hours	5 to 8 hours
Intermediate-acting	NPH	Humulin-N Novolin ge NPH	1 to 3 hours	5 to 8 hours	14 to 18 hours
Long-acting	detemir	Levemir	90 minutes	Virtually None	16 to 24 hours
	glargine	Lantus	90 minutes	None	24 hours
Premixed (the numbers after the names refer to the ratio of rapid- or short-acting insulin to intermediate-acting insulin)		Humalog Mix25 Humalog Mix50 Humulin (30/70) Novolin ge (30/70) NovoMix 30	Depends on specific type	Depends on specific type	Depends on specific type

One common misunderstanding is equating Humulin with Humulin-N. Humulin is a trade name and refers to a variety of types of insulin marketed by one particular company (Eli Lilly in this case). Humulin-N refers to Eli Lilly's brand of NPH insulin. To say you are on Humulin conveys the same degree of information as saying you drive a Chevrolet — helpful, but only part of the story. More specific would be if you said you drove a Malibu or an Impala or a Corvette. Even better would be if you said Ian could drive your Corvette!

You might notice in our discussions of the various types of insulin in this section that we mention basal-bolus insulin therapy a few times. *Basal-bolus insulin therapy* has, as you might guess, two components:

- **Basal insulin** (NPH, Levemir, Lantus): Insulin you give once (or, in some cases, twice) a day to prevent your blood glucose levels from climbing between meals.

- **Bolus insulin** (Apidra, Humalog, NovoRapid): Insulin you give before each meal to prevent your blood glucose levels from climbing after a meal. For this reason it is also referred to as mealtime insulin. (Although regular insulin can also be used as a bolus insulin, because it less closely replicates normal insulin release from the pancreas it is typically not as good a choice.)

The other way of using basal-bolus insulin therapy is with an insulin pump (see "How to Give Insulin" later in this chapter).

Basal-bolus insulin therapy forms the backbone (so to speak) of managing type 1 diabetes (and is also excellent therapy for many people with type 2 diabetes).

Basal-bolus insulin therapy is also commonly called *intensified insulin therapy.* Although we do use this term, we admit to not being overly fond of it, because *all* people with diabetes need to be treated intensively regardless of whether that means simply with diet and exercise, or oral hypoglycemic agents, or one, two, three, or more doses of insulin.

Assistance obtaining insulin

No one's health should suffer because they cannot obtain insulin due to financial hardship. If you require insulin therapy but have neither the money nor the insurance (governmental or private) coverage for it, you can still obtain insulin (without charge) in several ways.

You can contact the insulin manufacturers directly (all Canadian insulin manufacturers have compassionate care programs for this very purpose):

✔ Eli-Lilly (Lilly Canada Cares Insulin Assistance Program): 888-545-5972

✔ Novo Nordisk: 800-465-4334 (Novo Nordisk doesn't have a specific compassionate care program, but in special circumstances it will provide insulin to your doctor or diabetes educator who in turn can provide it to you.)

✔ Sanofi-Aventis (Lantus Compassionate Care Program): 800-265-7927

Additionally, try your diabetes educators. They will almost certainly have samples they can provide you with in a pinch.

Rapid-acting insulin

Three types of rapid-acting insulin are available: aspart (NovoRapid), lispro (Humalog), and glulisine (Apidra).

Rapid-acting insulin

> ✔ Is a mealtime insulin. That is, you take rapid-acting insulin to prevent your blood glucose levels from rising too high after your meal.

> ✔ Is a bolus component of basal-bolus insulin therapy.

> ✔ Can be taken anywhere between ¼ hour to immediately before you eat. (This will depend on how your blood glucose levels respond to the insulin. Some people get the best response taking it as long as ½ hour before a meal.)

> ✔ Has its peak effect at the same time as the glucose from your food is being absorbed from your small intestine, so the action of the insulin matches the rise in your blood glucose. That's what a healthy pancreas does, too.

✔ Wears off within a short period of time (three to five hours).

✔ Compared to regular insulin, is less likely to cause hypoglycemia, provides better after-meal blood glucose control, and is more convenient to use (it can be given as soon as immediately before a meal). As a result, rapid-acting insulin has largely replaced regular insulin in Canada.

If you have *gastroparesis* (a condition in which your stomach becomes less efficient at propelling food into your small intestine) *and* erratic blood glucose control, you may benefit from taking rapid-acting insulin an hour or so *after* your meal. Your diabetes specialist can help you determine if this would be a good option for you.

For all intents and purposes, all rapid-acting insulins are identical in their actions. Indeed, the only significant way in which they differ is that if you buy one type you help boost the share price of one company, and if you buy the other type you help the other company's valuation.

Regular insulin

Because regular insulin is sometimes referred to as a short-acting insulin (as in the Canadian Diabetes Association 2008 Clinical Practice Guidelines) and is sometimes referred to as a fast-acting insulin (as it was in the 2003 version of the Guidelines), you might get (understandably!) confused. For that reason, unless we forget, we refer to regular insulin as, simply, "regular insulin" throughout this book.

Regular insulin is also called Toronto insulin, but it is seldom called that anymore. (Too bad; it reminded people around the world of insulin's Canadian roots.)

These are the most important properties of this insulin. Regular insulin

✔ Is a mealtime insulin, given to prevent your blood glucose levels from rising too high after your meal.

✔ Is a bolus component of basal-bolus insulin therapy. (Although both regular insulin and rapid-acting insulin are bolus insulins, the latter is preferred, as we discuss in the preceding section.)

✔ Does not have much action until 30 minutes after you inject it, so you should take it — you guessed it — 30 minutes *before you eat.* That can be such a hassle, so most people end up taking it immediately before they eat anyhow. It'll still work, but not as effectively.

✔ Has a longer duration of action and is more likely to cause hypoglycemia than rapid-acting insulin.

✔ Is more likely to cause hypoglycemia, provides less effective after-meal blood glucose control, and is less convenient to use (as it needs to be given 30 minutes before a meal) than rapid-acting insulin. Consequently, doctors are recommending regular insulin less and less often.

Intermediate-acting insulin

NPH (sometime simply called *N*) is the only available intermediate-acting insulin. Intermediate-acting insulin

✔ Is given to prevent your blood glucose levels from going up too high between meals.

✔ Is a basal component of basal-bolus insulin therapy.

✔ Is often given at bedtime to prevent your blood glucose level from going up too high overnight. (We discuss this *dawn phenomenon* later in this chapter.)

✔ Does not have much effect until a few hours after it's injected, so it doesn't help to reduce your blood glucose levels immediately after you eat.

✔ Is more likely than long-acting insulin to cause hypoglycemia (including overnight). For this reason, NPH is being used less and less, and long-acting insulin more and more.

Long-acting insulin

Long-acting insulin works for, well, a long time. Two types of long-acting insulin are available: Levemir and Lantus. Long-acting insulins

✔ Are given to prevent your blood glucose levels from going up too high between meals.

✔ Are the basal component of basal-bolus insulin therapy.

✔ Are often given at bedtime to prevent your blood glucose level from going up too high overnight. (We discuss this dawn phenomenon later in this chapter.)

✔ Don't have a quick action, so they don't help to reduce your blood glucose levels immediately after you eat. For this reason, long-acting insulins are usually supplemented with rapid-acting (or regular) insulin given with meals (or, in the case of type 2 diabetes, sometimes with oral hypoglycemic agents).

✔ Have a very consistent action — they have pretty well the same effect on blood glucose levels two hours after the injection as they do eight or more hours after the injection. (Lantus has no peak action and Levemir has only a slight peak.)

✔ Last up to 24 hours, so they are typically taken just once per day. (There are, however, many exceptions to this pattern. Many people — particularly if taking Levemir, but also with Lantus — find they require it twice daily.)

✔ Result in more consistent blood glucose values (meaning that your blood glucose readings will be less variable) than with intermediate-acting insulin.

✔ Often cause less weight gain for those people newly starting insulin therapy than intermediate-acting insulin. (This may be particularly true of Levemir insulin.)

✔ Are less likely to cause hypoglycemia (including overnight) than intermediate-acting insulin. For this reason, long-acting insulins are being used increasingly often and intermediate-acting insulins less and less often.

✔ Should not be mixed in the same syringe with any other insulin.

✔ Cause discomfort in a small percentage of people upon injection. With Levemir insulin, an even smaller percentage may develop a sore, red rash at the injection site.

If you experience more than minimal discomfort when injecting these insulins or if you develop a rash at the injection site, be sure to promptly inform your physician because you may need to change the insulin to a different type.

✔ Cost much more than intermediate-acting insulin.

Levemir and Lantus insulins are clear (you can see through them). So are rapid-acting and regular insulins. Because of this similarity in appearance, people have mistakenly given themselves one type of insulin when they meant to give the other. Read the label very carefully before administering your insulin. (Because NPH insulin is cloudy, it isn't as likely to be confused with the other, clear types of insulin.)

Premixed insulin

Premixed insulin combines, in a single cartridge (or vial), both a mealtime insulin (either Humalog, NovoRapid, or regular insulin) and a longer-acting insulin (either NPH or another insulin that acts similar to it). The percentage of mealtime insulin and longer-acting insulin differs depending on the specific type of premixed insulin. Determining which of the various available premixed insulins provides the best blood glucose control for a given individual is largely a matter of trial and error. The various types of premixed insulin are listed in Table 3-1, earlier in the chapter.

If you ever need to buy premixed insulin in the United States, be aware that what we call 30/70 insulin here is called 70/30 insulin there.

The advantage of a premixed insulin is that you have to take it only twice per day (before breakfast and before supper). If you were to separately take bolus insulin (three injections per day) and basal insulin (one or two injections per day), you would need more frequent injections.

The huge disadvantage to premixed insulin is that, because it is premixed, you can't independently adjust each of its two insulin ingredients to match your body's specific requirements. Although some diabetes specialists use it often, we find premixed insulin seldom provides sufficient flexibility and blood glucose control, and therefore we don't routinely recommend it for people with type 2 diabetes and we never recommend it to people with type 1 diabetes.

Animal insulins

In very rare circumstances, people with diabetes are treated with animal insulins. The two available products are Hypurin Regular and Hypurin NPH, made by Wockhardt UK. You can find further information on this topic at www.hc-sc. gc.ca/dhp-mps/brgtherap/activit/fs-fi/qa_qr_ insulin_02_2006-eng.php. (Daunting task indeed to type this Web address into your browser; instead, just type the terms "Hypurin health Canada" into your Web search engine and this link to Health Canada's information on animal-sourced insulins will show up.)

Type 1 Diabetes and Insulin Therapy

The best insulin treatment strategy if you have type 1 diabetes is *basal-bolus* therapy, meaning that you either use an insulin pump (see "How to Give Insulin," later in this chapter) or you take intermediate- or long-acting (basal) insulin once (or twice) a day, and rapid-acting or regular (bolus) insulin prior to meals. Of these two methods, pump therapy is the best treatment currently available for type 1 diabetes because it most closely mimics what a normal pancreas does.

If you have type 1 diabetes and aren't being treated with basal-bolus therapy (with or without an insulin pump), contact your doctor to find out if you should change to one of these state-of-the-art forms of diabetes treatment.

Because Levemir and Lantus insulins, compared with NPH insulin, cause less hypoglycemia (including nocturnal hypoglycemia) and less blood glucose variability, they are often the preferred basal insulins for people with type 1 diabetes. On the other hand, long-acting insulins cost considerably more than NPH insulin. If you're doing well with NPH insulin as part of basal-bolus therapy, you don't *have to* change to Levemir or Lantus insulin. On the other hand, if you are having problems with overly frequent hypoglycemia (especially overnight) or inconsistent blood glucose readings, discuss with your doctor or diabetes educator switching from NPH to Levemir or Lantus.

Type 2 Diabetes and Insulin Therapy

Unfortunately, insulin therapy for people with type 2 diabetes has typically been looked at as a sign of failure, a last resort greeted with equal parts doom and gloom. What a shame! Insulin is simply one more treatment option — one that's terribly underused. Goodness knows how many people might have been spared complications if only insulin had been used sooner in the course of their therapy.

The right time for you to start insulin if you have type 2 diabetes is when you cannot achieve appropriate blood glucose control without insulin or when very quick blood glucose lowering is required (for example, if your blood glucose readings are very high and you are having symptoms from this). For some people that means starting insulin at the time of diagnosis; for others, after years of combined use of two or more oral hypoglycemic agents. The key point is that you and your health care team must always be looking at ways to optimize your glucose control. If lifestyle change does the trick, great. If oral agents bring your readings into target, terrific. What you want to avoid is the all-too-common scenario where the person with diabetes and their physicians spend month after month, year after year, awaiting a magical improvement in glucose control that simply isn't going to happen without insulin administration.

There is no "best" insulin to be on if you have type 2 diabetes; however, these strategies are particularly effective:

✔ Taking basal insulin (that is, NPH, Levemir, or Lantus) at bedtime and an oral hypoglycemic agent (particularly metformin; often in combination with a second oral hypoglycemic agent) during the daytime. This is our preferred way to begin insulin therapy for most insulin-requiring people with type 2 diabetes. The insulin (if given in sufficient dose) prevents blood glucose levels from rising unduly overnight, and the oral medications keep blood glucose levels under control during the day.

✓ Basal-bolus insulin therapy (see "Looking at the Types of Insulin" earlier in this chapter).

✓ Premixed insulin taken twice daily. (Because of the limited flexibility of this strategy, we use it less often.)

✓ Insulin pump therapy. (This is not often used to treat type 2 diabetes but is a good option for select people with this condition such as those who are very active, are lean, and who have not had a sufficient response to basal-bolus insulin therapy.)

Because metformin therapy complements the action of insulin for people with type 2 diabetes, it's typically used regardless of which of the aforementioned insulin strategies you follow.

Your diabetes educator, family physician, and diabetes specialist can help you decide which treatment program is best for you.

The importance of adherence to a program of proper nutrition and exercise should never be minimized. Doctors often see people who, despite being on huge doses of insulin and numerous oral hypoglycemic agent pills, are still having problems with glucose control — problems that improve virtually overnight when those people have made appropriate dietary changes and renewed efforts with exercise.

Debunking Insulin Myths

The longer we're in practice as diabetes specialists, the greater is our sadness when we meet patients who have developed diabetes complications that could have been avoided if only they had been made aware that certain beliefs they had about insulin therapy (and which led them to avoid it) were based on incorrect information. Well, in case you, too, have any misperceptions regarding insulin therapy, here we list a few of the most common insulin myths:

✓ **Giving insulin is difficult.** In fact, giving insulin is very, very simple and straightforward. And as a bonus, taking insulin often means you can discontinue a whole bunch of pills you might be presently (unsuccessfully) taking for blood glucose control.

✔ **Insulin needles hurt.** They are virtually pain free.

✔ **It's embarrassing to be seen giving an insulin injection.** With current techniques, such as using insulin pen devices, giving insulin is typically very discrete; indeed, the odds are good that you've sat near — or even right beside — someone in a restaurant who injected insulin and you never noticed.

✔ **Insulin will make me feel like I'm prisoner to my diabetes therapy.** Many people find taking insulin liberating as they discover how it allows greater flexibility (compared to some types of oral hypoglycemic agent they had been on prior to insulin) with meal timing, when they exercise, and so forth.

✔ **Insulin will make me feel unwell.** In fact, on insulin therapy you will likely feel *better* as your blood glucose levels improve — typically after many months (or even years) of suboptimal therapy on oral hypoglycemic agents that are no longer working sufficiently well for you.

✔ **Taking insulin means I've failed.** Taking insulin means your *pancreas* has failed, not you. Indeed, taking insulin means you've succeeded in adopting an excellent form of therapy.

✔ **Once you're on insulin, you're on it forever.** Insulin is used when your own pancreas can no longer sufficiently do its job. And because medical science doesn't have a way of making your pancreas rejuvenate itself, sure, most people who start insulin need to stay on it. But this isn't because insulin is addictive or creates dependency; it's because your underlying diabetes isn't going to go away. However, if you have type 2 diabetes and you're able to make appropriate lifestyle changes, including losing weight, then there is the chance that you could discontinue your insulin (under appropriate medical supervision) and replace it with oral hypoglycemic agent therapy.

✔ **Insulin leads to complications.** Perhaps your Aunt Sally went blind after she started insulin. If so, the insulin didn't cause it; in fact, the delay in starting insulin may have led to this.

> ✔ **Insulin will likely make me go into a coma.** Although taking insulin can lead to low blood glucose, which has the potential to cloud your thinking and even cause you to lose consciousness, this seldom happens to people with type 2 diabetes. And if you have type 1 diabetes, taking appropriate precautions will minimize this risk.

Insulin therapy has been improving and saving lives for over 80 years, yet it remains very underutilized, and as a result, many people get unnecessarily sick. We think that's a tragedy — and that's no myth.

Exploring Different Insulin Delivery Devices

There is, in truth, only one way to learn how to give yourself insulin, and that's by sitting down with a diabetes educator and having her or him teach you. You can no more learn how to give insulin by reading a package insert (or even this book, we're quite willing to admit) than you can learn how to drive a car without ever getting behind the wheel. This section will therefore address *general* principles of insulin administration.

Have you ever seen a movie where the actor says, "We can do this the easy way or we can do this the hard way. You decide." Well, the same applies to giving insulin.

You're an award winner

Two companies that manufacture insulin in Canada give out awards to celebrate those individuals who have used insulin for many years. NovoNordisk has the Novo Nordisk Half Century Award Program (recognizing, as you might surmise, 50 years of using insulin) and Eli Lilly has the Lilly Diabetes Journey Awards (of which there are three: one for 25 years of insulin use, one for 50 years of insulin use, and one for 75 years of insulin use). You can find out more about the Novo Nordisk award by calling 800-465-4334 and you can find out more about the Eli Lilly awards by calling 888-545-5972 or on the Web at www.lillydiabetes.com/content/lilly-programs.jsp (click on Journey Awards).

Pens and syringes

For decades, the only way to give insulin was with a syringe and a bottle. Giving insulin this way is perfectly acceptable. But so is driving a 1990 Chevy. It may get you where you want to go, but it isn't quite the same as driving a brand-new Lexus. By far the easiest way to inject insulin is with an insulin pen (see Figure 3-1). Pen devices are easy to use and are very reliable. The great majority of Canadians who use insulin give it with pen devices. Of the thousands of patients in Ian's practice, he can count the number of syringe users on the fingers of one hand.

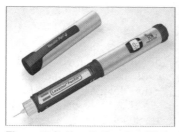 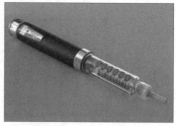

Figure 3-1: Novolin Pen 4 and HumaPen Luxura.

Here's what you need to know about insulin pens:

✔ Your diabetes educator or pharmacist can provide you with a free pen device.

✔ When you first start insulin, your diabetes educator will likely provide you with an initial, small, free supply of insulin for your pen device.

✔ Most pen devices are refillable. As your diabetes educator will demonstrate, you simply remove the used insulin cartridge and pop in a new one.

✔ Some pen devices are pre-filled with non-removable insulin cartridges. When they're used up, you return the entire pen to your pharmacy for appropriate disposal.

✔ Insulin pens have a display that tells you how much insulin you are about to inject. If your dose exceeds the maximal amount that can be delivered with one injection, you don't need to remove the needle and inject yourself again. Instead, you can re-dial the pen while the needle is still inserted.

Whether you've been taking insulin for 20 days or 20 years, a time may well come when you accidentally give yourself either the wrong insulin or the wrong dose, or even forget to give a dose altogether. Fortunately, such a slip-up seldom leads to anything serious. Don't feel guilty or stupid if you make a mistake with your insulin; it happens to everyone. The way to deal with this type of oversight will depend on many factors, including the type of insulin you are taking (or, ahem, not taking), the dose, your blood glucose control, and the type of diabetes you have. Because so many factors must be taken into account, it's best that you speak to your diabetes educator to formulate a plan of action if you make an error with your insulin.

Jet injectors

If neither pen devices nor syringes suit your fancy, and if you don't mind spending a whole bunch of money (about $700), you can obtain a jet injection device (such as the AdvantaJet Injector — www.advantajet.com — distributed in Canada by Activa Brand Products; 800-991-4464). The idea behind these is that because they don't have needles, using them to give insulin won't hurt as much. Although that's true for some people, it's not for others, and in any event, giving insulin with a pen device is virtually pain free anyhow. Jet injectors are rarely used in Canada.

Pumps

With each passing day, more and more Canadians with type 1 diabetes are changing from using insulin pens to insulin pumps. This is no surprise. Insulin pumps are reliable, effective, and sophisticated devices that are excellent tools to help manage diabetes. They are, however, definitely *not* the right choice for everyone.

Simply put, insulin pumps are pumps that pump insulin. They are the key component of what we call *continuous subcutaneous insulin infusion* (CSII) therapy. These are the basic components of CSII (see Figure 3-2):

✔ **An insulin pump:** These are small, pager-sized computer-ized devices with buttons that you press to program and instruct the pump on how much insulin to give you and when to give it.

✔ **An insulin reservoir** (which you fill with insulin every few days): The pump has a small motor that controls a cylinder that pushes the insulin from the reservoir into the attached tubing.

✔ **Tubing and insertion site:** The tubing carries the insu-lin from the pump to your body. It has two ends: One end connects to the reservoir on the pump and the other end connects to a tiny plastic needle that (using an inserter) you place just under the surface of the skin of your abdomen (or buttocks or arms or legs). The insulin reservoir, tubing, and insertion site are replaced every two to three days.

These are important aspects of pump therapy:

✔ Pump therapy is most suited to people with type 1 dia-betes who are on four or more insulin injections per day. People with type 2 diabetes who are on similar amounts of insulin may also benefit from pump therapy.

✔ An insulin pump uses only rapid-acting insulin. If you use pump therapy, you no longer administer insulin by syringe or pen and you no longer give intermediate- or long-acting insulin. Rapid-acting insulin most closely mimics insulin from a healthy pancreas.

✔ Just like a normal pancreas, the pump delivers small amounts of (basal) insulin into your body 24 hours a day. You must program the pump to tell it how much basal insulin to give.

✔ The pump, again like a normal pancreas, delivers extra (bolus) insulin into your body at mealtimes (and, often, with snacks). You must tell the pump — based on the type and amount of food you are about to eat — how much of this bolus insulin to give (typically, within 15 minutes prior to beginning your meal). For this reason, carbohydrate counting is a crucial element of successful pump management. (We discuss carbohydrate counting later in this chapter.)

✔ Pumps don't measure your blood glucose levels. If you use a pump, you must continue to do blood glucose meter tests. One pump is available in Canada (the MiniMed Paradigm REAL-Time Insulin Pump and Continuous Glucose Monitoring System) that combines an insulin pump with a glucose sensor to automatically measure and display your (interstitial fluid) glucose level, which in turn allows you to test your blood glucose level less frequently.

✔ Some pumps are said to be waterproof (indeed; some marathon swimmers successfully and uneventfully use these). Nonetheless, in general we feel it is best to avoid getting *any* pump wet (whether waterproof or not) in case its protective seal has been compromised, which could allow water to get into the pump and interfere with its function. Briefly disconnecting your pump while you take a dip (or shower) is usually a better option than swimming with it.

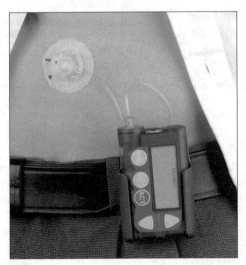

Figure 3-2: An insulin pump with its infusion set.

If you have diabetes, you already know that no aspect of treatment is perfect and that what is good for your next-door neighbour may not be good for you. This is true of pump therapy as well.

Here are the pros of pump therapy:

- ✓ **It's very convenient.** You have less stuff (syringes, vials, pens, needles, and so on) to carry around with you and it's much easier to bolus (that is, give an extra quantity of insulin) with meals and snacks. It also allows for much greater flexibility regarding meal timing, exercise, shift work, sleeping in, and other routine day-to-day aspects of your existence.

- ✓ **It provides better blood glucose control.** It can help smooth out blood glucose levels — with fewer episodes of hypo- and hyperglycemia — because problems with inconsistent and erratic insulin absorption of longer-acting insulins are no longer an issue. For many pump users, pump therapy also results in improved A1C readings.

These are pump therapy's cons:

- ✓ **It is *very* expensive.** A pump will cost you about $6,800, and supplies will run you about $250 per month (and that doesn't even include the cost of insulin or blood glucose test strips).

- ✓ **You and your pump are virtually inseparable.** You can disconnect your pump for an hour or so, such as when you shower or swim, but just like a teenager and a phone, separations must be kept to a minimum.

- ✓ **Pumps do not think for you.** They are clever computers, but they are still a darn sight less clever than your brain. You need to spend 15 or more hours being trained (by a "pump trainer" diabetes educator) how to operate and adjust your pump based on your glucose levels, your exercise, your diet, and so on. (Within the next few years this may change; rapid progress is being made on closing the loop, wherein a pump, in conjunction with a glucose sensor, would automatically know how much insulin to give you.)

- ✓ **It's lots of work.** If you aren't using a glucose sensor (we discuss these in Chapter 2), you must test your blood glucose 6 to 12 times per day, the pump's insulin infusion rate has to be frequently reassessed, you have to spend many hours with your diabetes educator to learn how to use your pump, and so on. If you aren't up to this type of commitment, then that nearly $7,000 insulin pump you just got will become nothing more than one very, very expensive paperweight.

Many private insurance companies (and, very recently, some provincial/territorial governments) will pay for most (or even all) of the cost of an insulin pump and supplies. Be sure to speak to them about this. They will likely require a supportive letter from your diabetes specialist and, in the case of governments, they will require that you meet a number of criteria. The pump companies themselves often offer interest-free financing as well as a several-month return policy so that if you decide you don't want to stay with a pump you can obtain a full refund. Be sure to find out all these details (in writing) before you commit yourself to a pump purchase.

When we first suggest pump therapy to our patients, the usual response we hear is, "Doctor, I can't imagine having that thing attached to me all the time. It would make me feel like a prisoner." But we must say that these words are seldom spoken by actual pump users; it's pretty well only people that haven't tried a pump who voice this concern. Indeed — and as surprising as this may seem — what we typically hear from our patients on insulin pumps is that they find pump therapy liberating and would never go back to conventional insulin injections. Heck, we'd have to wrestle them to the ground to get them to give up their pumps. And as for the extra work involved with pump therapy, that's a trade-off that pump users are invariably happy to make.

People often ask Ian why he is such a proponent of pump therapy. Ian replies that it is not just that the science shows it to be an excellent option (which it does), but also that his patients have convinced him. When patient after patient after patient tells Ian it's the best thing they've done since they were diagnosed with diabetes and they wished they'd done it sooner, this is not something that can be ignored. In Ian's opinion, for those people *who are appropriate candidates* and have the financial resources, pump therapy is not only the way of the future, it's the way of the present!

If you're trying to decide if a pump is for you — and, if it is, which pump to choose — your diabetes educator is the best person to speak with. Not all educators have studied pumps, so your educator may refer you to an even more specialized teacher called a "pump trainer." Speaking to pump users to hear what they have to say would also be a good idea. Your educator likely can provide you with the name of a "pumper" to contact (pump users are almost always more than happy to spread the word). You can also find more information on

Portrait of a pumper

Tom, a 24-year-old accountant, was a very active man and was exceptionally attentive to his diabetes management. He would test his blood five, six, seven, or more times per day and was giving himself Humalog insulin with meals and Levemir insulin at bedtime. In addition, when he snacked he would take a few extra units of Humalog. Some days he would take a total of seven injections of insulin. Tom's blood glucose readings and A1C were both excellent. "Tom," Ian said to him at the time of an appointment, "I think you should consider getting a pump." Tom was surprised and wondered why he should. "Because you are working very, very hard at managing your diabetes and I think you would find things are much easier for you on a pump," Ian replied. "Not easy, but easier."

Tom was hesitant at first but then decided to try the pump. A few months later he was back in the office. "How's it going?" Ian asked. "Well," Tom said, "I must admit I was a bit skeptical of your advice, but I decided to try the pump anyhow." Ian looked on expectantly. "And I have to tell you it was a fantastic decision. And like you said, life isn't now easy, but it is easier. When I need a bolus, presto, it's done. No one even notices when I give my insulin, not that that would bother me anyhow. And guess what; I'm having fewer lows than I was." Ian asked Tom if he would ever go back to his insulin pen injections. "Not on your life. They'd have to shoot me to get this pump from me!"

Tom was an ideal candidate for an insulin pump. He was testing and injecting many times per day. He was motivated and interested in putting in the considerable time and energy necessary to learn how to use a pump. In the absence of this devotion, switching to a pump is no more likely to make your glucose control better than driving a Porsche rather than a Hyundai instantly makes you a better driver.

pump therapy (and continuous glucose monitoring — see Chapter 2) by surfing over to a video on pump therapy that Ian made (www.drblumervideo.com) or by directly contacting the companies in Canada that sell insulin pumps:

- Animas Canada: www.animas.ca, 866-406-4844

- Medtronic Diabetes of Canada Ltd.: www.minimed.ca, 866-444-4649

- Roche Insulin Delivery Systems:
  www.accu-chekinsulinpumps-ca.com/dstrnc_ca, 800-280-7801

In our experience, we find that *all* the pumps currently available in Canada work very well. We also find that the pump companies provide excellent customer support. The decision to buy one brand of pump versus another, therefore, often comes down to which pump has a design you prefer, which display you like the best, and what other bells and whistles suit your fancy. The one other very important consideration is whether or not you want (or might want in the future) a pump that is integrated (or can be integrated) with a continuous glucose monitor (we discuss continuous glucose monitors in Chapter 2). If this last feature is important to you (and it is, appropriately, to most people), then your choices will be quickly narrowed down because only Medtronic presently offers such a combined device.

Caring for Your Insulin

Although insulin is not particularly difficult to look after, you should be aware of some handling issues:

- ✔ Do not use insulin after the expiration date marked on the label.

- ✔ Before its first use, store an *unopened* vial or cartridge of insulin in the refrigerator. (Refrigeration helps to preserve the potency of the insulin.)

- ✔ After you use it for the first time, you can keep your vial or cartridge of insulin either refrigerated or at room temperature (see the tip following this list).

- ✔ After its first use, your vial or cartridge of insulin has a limited time (usually about four weeks) before you will need to discard it. The package insert that came with your insulin will indicate the precise time recommended by the manufacturer of the particular insulin you are using.

- ✔ Insulin doesn't take well to excessive heat (such as being kept inside a car on a hot summer day) or, contrarily, to excessive cold (as Ian's patient found out when he returned to his car after his son's mid-winter hockey practice only to find his insulin bearing a surprising resemblance to a Popsicle). You should not use insulin that has been frozen or subjected to extreme heat.

✔ If you will be travelling to a destination where you won't have access to refrigeration facilities for insulin storage, use an insulated travel pack to keep your insulin protected from the elements. Frio (www.frious.com) makes a particularly good and quite novel line of travel packs that, when dunked in water, automatically start to cool. After a few days the cooling effect diminishes and it's time for another dunk.

✔ Many a person has successfully injected insulin through clothing, but we don't recommend you do it routinely.

✔ Most people reuse their needles, but because needles can get dull so quickly (which can both increase the discomfort of an injection and lead to skin damage including lipohypertrophy), we don't recommend doing this routinely either.

✔ Dispose of used needles in a puncture-proof "sharps" container that is sealed shut before being discarded. Most pharmacies will accept these containers and will dispose of them for you.

✔ If you're using cloudy insulin (some insulins are clear and some are cloudy), roll the vial to mix the contents before you inject it. If clumps are present, do not use the insulin.

You'll find that injecting insulin that is at room temperature is more comfortable than injecting insulin you have just taken out of the refrigerator.

Adjusting Your Insulin Dose

If you're taking insulin, you can pat yourself on the back; you have just been given the right to prescribe your own medicine. Well, not entirely, but to quite a significant extent. Insulin is different from almost any other medicine your doctor will ever ask you to take. Unlike antibiotics, heart medicines, or, for that matter, oral hypoglycemic agents, insulin is *not* designed to be taken in a set dose day to day. If your pancreas was working properly, it would constantly adjust how much insulin it was producing based on your body's requirements at any given moment. When you give yourself insulin, you're trying to mimic what your pancreas would normally do, so that means you, too, should be constantly adjusting your insulin dose. In fact, when we ask patients how much insulin they are taking, it is music to our ears when they reply, "Oh, well that depends. . . ." Precisely right. It depends. It depends on many things, including

- ✔ What you are about to eat (This refers to both the *type* of food — particularly the carbohydrate content — and the *amount* of food you're about to enjoy. We discuss the importance of *carbohydrate counting* if you have type 1 diabetes later in this chapter. Some people with type 2 diabetes also benefit from carbohydrate counting.)
- ✔ Your current blood glucose level
- ✔ Your recent blood glucose levels
- ✔ Whether you will be exercising
- ✔ Which type of insulin you are using

The common denominator in this list is the need to make *pro-active* insulin adjustments. The single greatest reason for failing to achieve good blood glucose control is making *retroactive* insulin adjustments. To be pro-active, you should be like a soothsayer, trying to predict what your reading is likely to be in a few hours and taking the amount of insulin *now* that will anticipate your needs *later*. Far too often people simply say, "Oh, my reading is high, I need more insulin," or "My reading is low, I need less insulin." These statements are perfectly true, but they take into account far less information than is available and necessary.

Although insulin adjustment is essential for the great majority of people with diabetes, if you have type 2 diabetes and have excellent blood glucose control on the same daily dose of insulin, it would not be necessary for you to make routine changes.

Many, many people have the mistaken impression that their insulin dose correlates to the severity of their diabetes. In case you're one of those people, we're glad you are reading this paragraph. Your insulin dose tells you (and us) absolutely nothing about how good or bad your diabetes is. You can be on 10 units per day and have all sorts of complications and difficulties with your diabetes, or you can be on 300 units per day and sail along very nicely, thank you very much. Just like you should wear the shoe size that your feet require, so should you take the dose of insulin your body requires. That's all there is to it.

Bill was a 65-year-old man with type 2 diabetes. He was taking 10 units of NPH insulin at bedtime. Although his readings were 5 to 7 mmol/L at bedtime, his before-breakfast blood glucose readings were running 10 to 12 mmol/L. Bill blamed the high readings on eating too big a bedtime snack, but when he reduced his snack, it didn't help. Ian suggested to Bill that he increase his bedtime insulin dose by one unit every night until his before-breakfast readings came down to target. Two weeks later, Bill was up to 24 units of insulin daily and his before-breakfast readings were down to 5 mmol/L.

Bill's problem is a very common one. In the absence of sufficient quantities of insulin in your system, your blood glucose level will tend to rise overnight as your liver starts to release glucose into the blood (starting at about 3 a.m.) in response to increasing levels of other hormones (such as cortisol and growth hormone). This is called the *dawn phenomenon.* Intermediate- or long-acting insulin (the former routinely taken at bedtime; the latter usually but not always taken at bedtime) is the ideal way to combat this as the insulin will provide a substantial effect in the middle of the night to combat the liver's tendency at that time to release glucose. To get this benefit from your insulin, however, the dose *has to be adjusted* to meet your body's demands, as Bill discovered.

If you have elevated before-breakfast readings, but you are also having lows in the middle of the night, then you should *not* increase your bedtime insulin. The best solution will depend on what insulin you're taking. If you're having overnight hypoglycemia, we recommend, in consultation with your doctor and diabetes educator, the following options to help you avoid this problem:

- ✔ If you're taking NPH insulin at suppertime, change the time you take it to bedtime.

- ✔ If you're taking regular insulin at suppertime, discontinue this and take a rapid-acting insulin at suppertime instead.

- ✔ If you're taking NPH at bedtime, discontinue this and take Levemir or Lantus instead.

- ✔ If you're taking Levemir or Lantus at bedtime, reduce the dose. If that doesn't help, take it earlier in the day.

For generations, health care providers and people with diabetes have believed that high blood glucose readings first thing in the morning were sometimes (or often) a rebound from having had (and slept through) a low in the middle of the night. (This is called the *Somogyi phenomenon* or a *Somogyi reaction.*) With the introduction of continuous glucose monitoring (see Chapter 2), we now know that this type of rebounding seldom, if ever, occurs. So if you have a high blood glucose reading when you wake up in the morning, it's much more likely that your glucose levels have been steadily creeping up overnight; not that they were low (but you were unaware of it) in the middle of the night. The best way to be sure about what's going on is, from time to time, for you to set your alarm for the middle of the night and get up and test your blood glucose at that time.

When you start insulin, you must consider it as just that, *a start.* You'll need to stay in regular touch with your diabetes educator for *ongoing* dosage adjustment guidance. Your educator knows you as an individual and can provide advice specific to you. For example, your educator will help you learn how to adjust your doses based on your blood glucose readings, your diet, your exercise, your travelling, and, for women, where you are in your menstrual cycle. Without the educator's ongoing assistance, very few people ever master insulin adjustment and they typically end up feeling very frustrated. You may find it helpful to have a look at a handout Ian gives his patients who are about to start insulin (www.ourdiabetes.com/insulin-initiation.htm).

Carbohydrate Counting

Carbohydrates are *the* key nutrient in raising blood glucose readings after meals. You can take advantage of this by adjusting your insulin dose to fit with the likely effect on your blood glucose of the quantity of carbohydrates you are about to eat. This is called *carbohydrate counting* (*carb counting* for short) and is an essential part of type 1 diabetes management, especially if you're using an insulin pump. It can also be a helpful component of type 2 diabetes management if you're taking rapid-acting insulin with your meals.

The best way to learn how to perform carbohydrate counting is by meeting with your registered dietitian. They are expertly trained in this field and will likely spend at least an hour with you to go over the basics. Having a follow-up meeting (or meetings) with them to have the principles of carb counting reinforced is often a good idea.

Mary was a 16-year-old girl with type 1 diabetes. She was taking Lantus insulin at bedtime (to prevent her blood glucose from rising overnight) and was taking Humalog insulin with each meal to prevent her blood glucose readings from climbing too high after she ate. Nonetheless, she found that sometimes her two-hour, after-meal readings were excellent and other times they were poor, without any rhyme or reason. Mary met with the registered dietitian and discovered there was indeed a reason: Her consumption of carbohydrate was varying quite a bit from meal to meal, but she wasn't adjusting her insulin dose. Mary learned how to adjust her insulin based on how much carbohydrate she was eating, and soon thereafter her readings were excellent.

The first step in carbohydrate counting is to calculate how many grams of carbohydrate you're about to consume and to then give a certain number of units of rapid-acting insulin based on that. (See the following tip.) Because each person responds differently, adults are typically arbitrarily started on a ratio of 1 unit of insulin for every 10 grams of carbohydrate, but it can range from 1 unit per 5 grams to 1 unit per 20 grams. (And even that's not written in stone.) Bear in mind that not all carbohydrates will raise your blood glucose to the same degree. Do not count the fibre you eat when totalling the number of carbs in your diet because, although it's a carbohydrate, it will not raise your blood glucose.

You can find out the carbohydrate (including fibre) content of foods by having a look at the Nutrition Facts label on the food you buy. Also, some excellent books are available to help you learn and use carb counting. One particularly helpful book is *The Calorie King Calorie, Fat & Carbohydrate Counter* (Family Health). Also, some so-called smart insulin pumps are smart indeed and can perform the required calculations for you; all you have to do is tell the pump how many grams of carbs you're about to eat (and some of these devices make even that step easier by coming with a pre-loaded inventory of foods and their carbohydrate content). Bon appétit!

Having a honeymoon — whether or not you're married

The *honeymoon period* is a period of time after the onset of type 1 diabetes when individuals have some recovery of their pancreatic function and are able to stop giving themselves insulin injections (or, at least, require far lower doses than they had been on). Typically this lasts for no more than a few weeks or months. All honeymoons are short, including — with rare exceptions — this one.

If you're carbohydrate counting, you'll also benefit from using a *correction factor* (or *insulin sensitivity factor*). A correction factor tells you the amount of insulin you'll need to bring an elevated before-meal blood glucose level down to normal. In other words, your correction factor corrects your elevated blood glucose (and your carb counting–determined dose prevents your level from going up from the food you're about to eat).

Yolanda has type 1 diabetes treated with Humalog insulin with meals and Levemir insulin at bedtime. She's about to eat supper. Her before-supper blood glucose is 12 mmol/L. Her about-to-be-devoured scrumptious meal contains 40 grams of carbohydrate. She uses a carbohydrate counting ratio of 1 unit per 10 grams of carbohydrate (a 1:10 ratio) and a correction factor of 1 unit for each 5 mmol/L her blood glucose is above 7. To know how much insulin she needs to take, she does the following calculation:

1. She uses her carbohydrate counting ratio: 40 g of carbohydrate × 1 unit/10 g = 4 units

2. She uses her correction factor: 12 mmol/L – 7 mmol/L = 5 mmol/L × 1 unit/5 mmol/L = 1 unit

3. She adds these two amounts together and determines she needs 4 units + 1 unit = 5 units.

4. She injects 5 units of insulin and smiles to herself as she recalls how the once intimidating notion of carb counting and use of a correction factor came quickly to seem like second nature after she had spent an hour with the wonderful dietitian.

Donating blood

If you're on insulin therapy, Canadian Blood Services' current policy is that you are not a candidate to give blood. We are sure this policy is well intentioned, but we feel it's overly restrictive. (Incidentally, the American Red Cross allows people being treated with insulin to donate blood so long as they have never taken *beef* insulin.) If you are on oral hypoglycemic agents, you are eligible to donate blood unless some other health problem precludes this.

Carbohydrate counting may not be rocket science, but it isn't easy either and it's certainly not for everyone. If you're doing very well without carbohydrate counting, don't feel you have to take on this additional task. If, however, things aren't going sufficiently well for you (and in particular if your glucose control is inconsistent and/or your A1C isn't particularly good), you should contact your dietitian to discuss whether carbohydrate counting would be good for you.

Travelling with Your Insulin

We live in a mobile society, and if you use insulin, then where you go, your insulin goes too.

Breezing through the border

As you well know, airline security is now greater than ever. And this means you will need to take some additional measures when you are planning on travelling by plane.

The Canadian Air Transport Security Authority has issued guidelines for when you are flying with diabetes supplies. The following information is from the Canadian Diabetes Association's reference to these guidelines:

> ✔ Advise the security personnel that you have diabetes and that you're carrying your supplies on board. Have available a letter from your physician indicating that you have diabetes and that you need to carry your diabetes medication and supplies.

✔ Organize your medication and supplies into one separate container and take it with you in your *carry-on* (not your stowed) baggage.

✔ Ensure that your syringes have the needle guards in place and are accompanied by the insulin.

✔ Place your insulin and any other medications in a container with a professionally printed pharmaceutical label identifying the medication. If the pharmaceutical label is on the outside of the box containing the insulin, the insulin must be carried in that original packaging.

✔ Cap your lancets. They must be accompanied by a glucose meter imprinted with the manufacturer's name.

✔ If you have any difficulty throughout the screening process, request to speak to the screening supervisor.

✔ If you are travelling outside of Canada, consult with your airline for applicable international regulations.

If you use an insulin pump, you may wish to pre-emptively notify the screening officer that you are wearing the device. They will probably not bat an eye (insulin pumps are quickly becoming so commonplace they are likely seeing them routinely), but it may spare you some additional time and questions.

An insulin pump–wearing patient of Ian's was recently passing through airport security in an Asian country when the screener yanked her out of line. The patient surmised that the screener was alarmed by the presence of an unfamiliar device. Wrong! The screener smiled broadly as he lifted up his shirt to show Ian's patient that he, too, was a pump user! He then let her continue her otherwise uneventful journey through security.

There are at least three important reasons to take your insulin and supplies (injection devices, blood glucose meter, lancets, and so on) with you as part of your carry-on (not your checked) luggage:

✔ If you are going to Sydney, Nova Scotia, for example, your *carry-on* luggage is not going to get mistakenly sent to Sydney, Australia.

✔ The baggage compartment temperatures may not be appropriate for your insulin.

✔ You will need it!

And although not technically an insulin supply, make sure you take extra snacks with you on board in case your meals are delayed.

And on the subject of insulin supplies, if you will be travelling for any sort of extended period, make sure you have lots of extra insulin, blood glucose test strips, and so on. Better to have too much than to try finding a pharmacy at midnight in an unfamiliar city.

The Canadian Diabetes Association offers travel insurance to its members.

Because rapid-acting insulin works so quickly, even if you see the flight attendant moving the food cart down the aisle in your direction, do *not* take your insulin dose until your food has been set down in front of you. We've had more than one patient who, anticipating imminent arrival of his meal, took his rapid-acting insulin only to find the food cart then quickly whisked away when unexpected turbulence interrupted food services. With his mealtime insulin having been given but no meal to go with it, he was at risk of having hypoglycemia. Fortunately, he had wisely taken some snacks with him in his carry-on luggage and substituted the snacks for the missed meal.

Adjusting your doses between time zones

Travelling seldom causes big problems, especially if you're on basal-bolus therapy (we define this earlier in this chapter). Often the best thing to do is to

- ✔ Take your *bolus* insulin at your new mealtimes, regardless of when they happen to be.

- ✔ Take your *basal* insulin at the same hour of the clock you normally take it. For example, if you live in Vancouver and usually take, say, Lantus insulin at 10 p.m. *PST* and you then travel to Montreal — which has a three-hour time difference — you would instead take your Lantus insulin at 10 p.m. *EST*. The first day you would end up taking your injection three hours earlier than usual (and, upon your return, three hours later than usual), but this is seldom a problem with basal insulins. Thereafter you would be taking your basal insulin every 24 hours as you likely do customarily.

If there is going to be a significant delay between meals, take a snack and a small amount of your rapid-acting or regular insulin halfway between those meals.

 If your travels will take you beyond more than a few time zones or if you are not taking basal-bolus insulin, we recommend that you be in touch with your diabetes educator before you travel to get advice specific to your situation. Bon voyage!

Was inhaled insulin just so much hot air?

For years, the diabetes world was awaiting the development and availability of inhaled insulin. Many companies were working feverishly to develop such a product as they anticipated a financial windfall. Well, billions upon billions of research and development dollars later, inhaled insulin has come . . . and gone. Pfizer Corporation launched Exubera in the United States in 2006, then, quicker than Harry Potter can say "expelliarmus," withdrew it from the market citing poor sales. Seems like Exubera sales were anything but exuberant. Quickly following suit, pretty well every other company developing inhaled insulin — with the notable exception of Mannkind Corporation — halted their own initiatives to develop similar products.

However, other, novel routes of insulin administration continue to be explored. The Canadian company Generex Biotechnology Corporation has developed Oral-lyn, an aerosol form of insulin that is sprayed onto the inside of the cheek. It's now available for use in Ecuador and India. Whether it will prove to be a safe, effective, and useful product remains to be seen.

Chapter 4

Ten Ways to Stay Healthy and Avoid Complications

● ●

In This Chapter

▶ Learning for life

▶ Living healthfully

▶ Monitoring your numbers

▶ Keeping an eye on your vision and your feet

▶ Mastering your medicines

● ●

*W*e're thrilled you're reading this chapter because here we discuss the top ten things you need to know to stay healthy with your diabetes. If we were given a podium high enough and a speaker loud enough, these are the key messages we would shout out for all to hear.

If you don't have diabetes yourself and are reading this book on behalf of someone you love who does (which many of our readers tell us is the case), even if your loved one elects not to read this book in its entirety, please insist he or she looks at this chapter. Blame us for your insistence.

Following the advice on these pages could be the difference between disability and early death or a long and healthy life. More than two-thirds of diabetes complications are avoidable if the ten points we discuss in this chapter are followed. We consider it a tragedy, one that frustrates us and saddens us to the point of tears, that people are getting sick and even dying because they don't know the information in this chapter. We wrote this book — and particularly this chapter — to change things.

The ten points we discuss in this chapter are, indeed, the ten most important ways that you can stay healthy and lead a full and active life with your diabetes. And these measures are readily available to each and every person with diabetes. But — and this is a very big but — remember one other crucial point: Even if you follow just a portion of the recommendations in this chapter, you're still making headway. Even if you don't meet all your targets for weight control, blood glucose, blood pressure, and so forth, that doesn't mean you've failed and it doesn't mean it was all for naught. Any improvement in your weight or exercise or blood pressure or glucose levels or any of the other items we list here will help you reduce your likelihood of developing complications. So be proud of your work and your successes and, for those things lagging behind, well, it's always good to have additional goals to strive for.

Learn for Life

Every day, the two of us read professional journals or attend lectures or go to conferences, all with the express purpose of educating ourselves about how best to look after people with diabetes. And the family physicians we work with do the same. As do the diabetes nurse educators and dietitians. As do the podiatrists and the pharmacists and all the other professionals whose mission is to help you stay healthy. Your whole diabetes team is always learning. You, too, are a part of your diabetes team. So that means you also have to do your share of leaning.

The more you know, the better your odds are of being healthy. Ian's motto — present on the home page of his Web site (www.ourdiabetes.com) and guiding his professional life — is the saying, "Rule your diabetes; don't let it rule you!" Your continued education is the single most important factor in allowing you to do this. Don't be in the dark. Know what you should eat. Know how you should exercise. Know what your blood pressure is and what it should be, what your lipids are and what you are aiming for. Know what the best medicines are and how to safely and effectively use them. Whoever said "Ignorance is bliss" surely didn't have diabetes. Or, if they did, they likely came to rue the day they said it.

Don't be a passive partner in your diabetes care; be actively involved. You can learn from the other members of your health care team (especially from your diabetes nurse educator and dietitian). You can learn by reading this book (and the full version of *Diabetes For Canadians For Dummies*), reviewing (reputable) Web sites such as that of the Canadian Diabetes Association (www.diabetes.ca), and attending meetings of your local CDA branch. Until there is a cure for diabetes, learning needs to be a part of your life. It's as simple as that.

Remember that you'll find a lot of misinformation on the Web, so you must be careful to check out a recommendation before you start to follow it. Even information on reliable sites may not be right for your particular problem.

Eat Earnestly

The most important point about a "diabetic diet" is that it is a healthy diet for anyone, with diabetes or without. You shouldn't feel like a social outcast because you're eating the right foods. And you shouldn't feel guilty if occasionally you eat the wrong foods either, for that matter. **Remember:** There is no such thing as cheating. A healthy diabetes meal plan is not a crash diet, a high-protein diet, a grapefruit diet, or any other fad diet. A diabetes meal plan is a lifelong program of healthy, well-balanced eating.

You can follow a diabetes meal plan wherever you are, not just at home. Every menu has something on it that's appropriate for you. If you're invited to someone's home, let them know you have diabetes and that you can eat only a limited amount of carbohydrate and fat. If that fails, then limit the amount that you eat. And if that's somehow not possible, then accept the fact that your diet won't always be perfect (and whose is?) and go on from there.

Follow a healthy diet designed by both you and your dietitian and you'll have an excellent foundation in your plan for good health. Ignore proper nutrition and you'll be destined to have poor glucose control; indeed, both the pills and the insulins we use to control blood glucose are much less effective in the absence of a proper diet. Your destiny is in your hands — and in your mouth.

If you're looking for more information about eating right, check out the simply delicious *Diabetes Cookbook For Canadians For Dummies*, co-written by Ian with Cynthia Payne (Wiley).

Exercise Enthusiastically

If we were to tell you that we had a treatment for you to take that would cost you nothing; that would only have to be taken once per day; that could help keep your blood glucose levels under control, reduce your blood pressure, improve your lipids, reduce your stress level, and help prevent heart attacks; and that could lower your risk of dying over the next ten years by one-half, you would not only be wanting it, you would be demanding it! Okay then, it's yours. Exercise.

Preferably daily (or at least most days of the week). Preferably for at least 30 minutes per day. Make exercise as much a part of your life as breathing. The key to success with exercise? Finding the type you like and sticking with it. There is no need to run the Boston Marathon or swim across Lake Ontario (though you are welcome to if you want); something as simple (and inexpensive) as a daily walk is highly therapeutic.

Give the Heave-Ho to Harmful Habits

You win a lottery . . . but lose your ticket. You buy a brand-new car . . . and minutes later, lock your keys inside. You have a breakaway . . . and mishandle the puck. We all have our missteps — golden opportunities that we manage to make a mess of. But most of these are small miscues or, at worst, temporary setbacks. Having diabetes may be no piece of cake (well, actually, you can have a piece of cake, but that's another story), but with careful management you can lead a full, active, and long life. What a shame that smoking can wreck all that.

Smoking is bad enough for a person without diabetes, but if you have diabetes, smoking makes almost every complication more likely to occur. In essence, smoking rots your arteries.

You place yourself at enormous risk of a heart attack or a stroke, blindness, or amputations; the list goes on and on. But you can change the odds. Quit smoking now and you can markedly improve your likelihood of avoiding these complications. Some things in life are beyond our control. Smoking isn't one of them. Millions of Canadians have quit smoking. So can you.

Does it seem unfair that once you were diagnosed as having diabetes, all those well-meaning people (family, friends, doctors, nurses, dietitians, . . .) asked you to change your diet, your exercise, your weight, and, if you smoke, your tobacco use too? Well, if you think so, then you may also think it unfair that we will now ask you to moderate your drinking. No more than one (for women) or two (for men) a day. Tops. Your health is our raison d'être. No apologies for that.

Controlling Your Numbers: Optimizing Your Blood Glucose, Blood Pressure, Cholesterol, and Kidney Function

You can rest assured that your doctor knows your average blood glucose (as reflected by your A1C level), your blood pressure, your cholesterol, and your kidney function. Yet despite this, most Canadians with diabetes don't have all these levels under control and as a result are developing what are often avoidable complications. Clearly something's wrong with this picture.

We won't go into all the many factors here, but will point out one particularly important and easily correctable one: Most people with diabetes don't know their own numbers, and as a result don't know when they are above target (we discuss targets in the following sections), and thus, also don't know when corrective action needs to be taken.

"If it ain't broke, don't fix it," some people say. Okay, we'll go along with that. But what if you don't know that it's broke? What then? Your blood glucose, blood pressure, cholesterol, and kidney function tests all belong to *you*. Indeed, they're part of you. And you need to know them. Period.

Now that we've hopefully convinced you (perhaps you didn't need convincing), let's look at the numbers you should be targeting and what to do if they are being exceeded.

Blood glucose levels

High blood glucose is a toxin to your body. It can lead to blindness, kidney failure, and nerve damage. But you're clearly not just waiting around for bad things to happen; if you were, you wouldn't be reading this book right now. To prevent high blood glucose from damaging your body, be sure to test your blood glucose regularly. (Refer to Chapter 2.) Your blood glucose target is 4 to 7 mmol/L before meals, 5 to 10 mmol/L two hours after meals. Your A1C target is no more than 7. If your A1C is above 7 despite good before-meal readings, then your two-hour, after-meal target is 5 to 8 mmol/L. (These are the targets for the great majority of people with diabetes. Target values are different for children, pregnant women, and some elderly individuals.)

If your blood glucose levels are too high, speak to your health care team (particularly your diabetes nurse educator, dietitian, family doctor, and, if you have one, your diabetes specialist) about what changes can be made to your treatment plan to help get your blood glucose control where it should be.

Lipids (cholesterol and triglycerides)

High LDL cholesterol, low HDL cholesterol, high triglycerides, and a high total cholesterol/HDL ratio are bad things. Low LDL, high HDL, low triglycerides, and a low total cholesterol/ HDL ratio are good things. Now, which package do you want for your birthday? Got the wrong gift? So trade it in. Don't accept poor lipids. Optimal lipids will reduce your risk of cardiovascular disease, so optimal lipids are what we're after. The CDA target is for the LDL level to be less than or equal to 2 mmol/L and the total cholesterol/HDL ratio to be less than 4. These are the priorities. Be sure to know your own levels, and, if they are above target, speak to your physician to discuss how to make things better. She may recommend a visit to the dietitian, a change to your exercise program, or medication.

Blood pressure

Among the nasty things that high blood pressure causes are strokes, eye damage, heart attacks, and kidney failure. Quick: What was your blood pressure the last time your doctor checked it? And was that within the CDA target? If you know these two answers, congratulations. If you don't, then we're again thrilled that you're reading this. Your blood pressure should be less than 130/80. If your value is higher than this, speak to your doctor about how you can bring it into target.

See Your Eye Doctor

You may have 20/20 vision; heck, you may be able to see a speck of dust on the back of a gnat on the tail of a bird on the top of a tree on the peak of a mountain — but what you can't see is the back of your eyes. Only a skilled eye professional can determine the true health of your eyes. Don't be misled into thinking that your visual acuity (as reflected by your need for — and the strength of — prescription lenses) has anything to do with the health of your eyes. It doesn't. See your eye doctor regularly so you can, well, continue to see your eye doctor.

Fuss Over Your Feet

We walk, on average, about 184,000 kilometres in our lifetime. That's over four trips around the equator (well, okay, we realize that those darn oceans would keep getting in the way, but you know what we mean). So if you want to keep those lovely lower appendages of yours up to this task, you gotta look after 'em. Having diabetes means that your feet are at risk of damage including ulcerations, infections, and even frank gangrene and, potentially, amputation. But these devastating complications are largely avoidable. Go ahead, love your feet. It's okay; really. In fact, it's essential.

Master Your Medicines

You may have noticed that your success with diabetes is based on a combination of things, including knowledge, lifestyle treatment, and medicine use. Although no one wants to take medicines, you cannot underestimate their importance. Indeed, with each passing year, physicians are asking people with diabetes to take more and more pills. The reason is simple: These medicines can keep you healthy and even save your life. Most people with diabetes need to take medicines to accomplish one or more of the following:

- **Optimize blood glucose:** If you have type 2 diabetes, this usually requires metformin, often with one or two other blood-glucose-lowering medicines.

- **Optimize blood pressure:** This usually requires an ACE inhibitor or ARB along with one, two, or even three other types of medicine.

- **Optimize lipids:** This usually requires a statin and sometimes another medicine as well.

- **Prevent heart attacks and strokes:** If you're at high risk of cardiovascular disease, you should be taking either an ACE inhibitor or an ARB.

- **Prevent kidney failure:** If you have any evidence of diabetes-related kidney malfunction, you should be taking an ACE inhibitor or ARB.

- **Prevent pneumonia:** (At least this isn't a pill you have to remember to take!) Many people with diabetes fall ill each year from pneumonia. But you can markedly reduce your risk for developing influenza pneumonia by the simplest of measures: Have an annual flu shot. You should also have a vaccination to protect you against a different form of pneumonia called pneumococcal pneumonia (revaccination is sometimes given five years after the initial vaccination).

More controversial is whether or not people with diabetes should routinely take ASA to prevent blood clots.

"My goodness!" you might (and should) say. "That could be seven or more different types of medicine to take every day." No one should tell you that's not a big deal. It *is* a big deal. But lying in a hospital bed with a stroke or an amputation or a dialysis machine at your side is, by far, a bigger deal. We have the means to keep you healthy and to help you live a long, full life. And those means include medicines. Don't think of the pills you need to swallow each day as an anchor dragging you down. Think of them as a life preserver lifting you up!

Help Your Doctor Help You

Your family doctor went through four years of undergraduate university then four years of medical school then two or more years of further training for one simple reason: Your doctor is a glutton for punishment. (Please don't tell your doctor we said that! We really, really didn't mean it.)

Your doctor did all this training because he wanted to be suitably equipped to help you stay healthy. But without your help, all that training is largely wasted. Having diabetes is not like having appendicitis. If you have appendicitis, all you have to do is lie on an operating table while the anesthetist puts you to sleep and the surgeon takes out your diseased organ. If you have diabetes, on the other hand, you have to be an active and keen partner, working with your doctor by regularly attending appointments, sharing with your doctor how you are doing with your nutrition program and your exercise, what your blood glucose levels are, what your blood pressure is (when, for example, using a machine at a drugstore), if you are missing doses of your medicines or believe you're having side effects from them, and if you're experiencing symptoms such as chest pain or shortness of breath, erectile dysfunction or vaginal discharge, numbness or burning in your feet, and so on.

Your doctor relies on you to work with her for the common goal of keeping you healthy. Without your help, your doctor may just as well take those diplomas down off the wall and burn them. And that we do truly mean.

Don't Try to Do It Alone

In the previous section we discuss how you and your doctor can successfully work together. Many other health care professionals, including diabetes nurse educators and dietitians, podiatrists, eye specialists, pharmacists, and others, are not only available to help you, but are keen to help you. Also, never underestimate the importance of your *family's* involvement on your health care team. If someone else in the home does the cooking, take him or her with you when you meet with the dietitian. Have family members learn how to help you if your blood glucose level is low. If you can't inspect your own feet, ask a loved one to look for you. And if, at times, you're feeling frustrated or even fed up with the hassles of living with diabetes from day to day (we'd never deny that having diabetes can be a hassle), seeking the comfort of a loved one is often the best medicine of all.

Chapter 5

Ten Frequently Asked Questions

*T*hough every person with diabetes is unique — and needs to be treated as such — some questions do come up remarkably often. Sometimes it's because the answer isn't obvious (for instance, why in the world blood glucose levels would go up overnight even if you haven't been eating), and sometimes it's because the answer isn't easy to find (for example, how to get your doctor to be a more effective communicator). This chapter looks at the ten most commonly asked questions that we hear in our offices. (And we even supply the answers!)

Why Are My Blood Glucose Levels Higher When I Get Up in the Morning than When I Go to Bed?

Those higher blood glucose levels in the morning can seem like quite a conundrum. Did you take an unremembered stroll to the fridge at 3 a.m.? Not likely, unless you're one very hungry sleepwalker. Was it an overly big snack at bedtime that made your readings go up? Improbable, unless your snack was so huge that it would make Dagwood Bumstead proud. No, the answer lies within your body, not within your fridge or pantry.

Beginning about 3 a.m., your body starts to increase production of hormones such as cortisol and growth hormone, which are important for normal metabolism but which can, in a person with diabetes, lead to the release of glucose from the liver. This is called the *dawn phenomenon.*

Although this is a common problem, it's not one we take, ahem, lying down. The most successful strategy to fight the dawn phenomenon is to take a dose of intermediate- (NPH) or long-acting (Lantus, Levemir) insulin at bedtime. (Sometimes Lantus and Levemir are given at other times.) Suppertime doses of some oral hypoglycemic agents such as metformin or glyburide can also help but are often less effective.

If you're having this problem despite already taking bedtime insulin, then a simple solution may be to increase your insulin dose. Be sure to discuss this possibility with your physician or diabetes educator.

We discuss insulin issues in detail in Chapter 3.

Why Are My Blood Glucose Levels All Over the Place?

If you're like most people with diabetes (especially type 1 diabetes), you will have experienced times when, despite your best efforts, your glucose control seemed a mess. High one minute, low the next. High for a couple of days, low for the next two. Up and down, down and up, for no apparent rhyme or reason.

But of course there's a reason; there's *always* a reason. It's just a matter of detective work to figure out what that reason is. Sometimes doctors and patients naively think that all we have to worry about in terms of glucose control is what you eat, how you exercise, and what medicines you take. Although these are the most important factors, many other things can influence blood glucose control, including your stress level, your stomach and bowel function, your menstrual cycle, and more.

We discuss these issues in detail in Chapter 2.

Why Are My Blood Glucose Levels Getting Worse as Time Goes By?

Few things are as frustrating to a person with type 2 diabetes as finding that, despite following a proper diet (with occasional indiscretion — which is perfectly fine, by the way), taking more and more pills, and exercising regularly (okay, maybe irregularly, but doing some anyhow), his or her blood glucose levels are progressively worsening. If you have been in this situation, you probably asked yourself, "What am I doing wrong?"

The answer is, you are probably doing nothing wrong.

The problem is that diabetes is a progressive disease. We wish it wasn't, but it is. Which means that despite your (and our) best efforts, your pancreas is going to have a hard time keeping up. In fact, the day your type 2 diabetes was diagnosed, your pancreas was already running at only half normal function, and with each passing year it's likely to lose more and more of its ability to produce insulin. The net result is that, with all likelihood, you're going to require more and more medicine to control your glucose levels as time goes by. Worsening pancreas function is also the reason that the majority of people with type 2 diabetes will eventually require insulin therapy. That's not a sign that *you* have failed; it's a sign that *your pancreas* has. And that, of course, is not your fault.

It's theoretically possible that certain types of medicine will help slow down (or even stop) this deterioration in pancreas function. We have some evidence that TZD drugs may help preserve the pancreas's function, but if so, it's only to a limited extent. Newer incretin-based therapies also may help to protect the pancreas, but this is not yet proven. Stay tuned. . . .

What's the Difference between an A1C Level and a Blood Glucose Level?

One of the most important tests in assessing overall glucose control is also one of the least understood. Your A1C (hemoglobin A1C) helps us know what your average blood glucose level has been over the preceding three months. It's measured in percentage (unlike blood glucose, which is measured in mmol/L), and the result represents the proportion of your hemoglobin (the substance in your red blood cells that carries oxygen) that's permanently attached to glucose. The higher your average glucose readings over the preceding few months, the more glucose your hemoglobin is exposed to and the higher your A1C will be. Because it's an entirely different test from the one for blood glucose level, an A1C of 7 percent, for example, does not mean that your average blood glucose level is 7 mmol/L, but, rather, indicates your average blood glucose is 8.6 mmol/L. Fortunately, on the near horizon we will likely abandon discussing average blood glucose in terms of A1C levels and instead will simply use the same units (mmol/L) that you measure when doing your blood glucose meter tests. This will surely make life easier for both people with diabetes and health care professionals alike.

We discuss this in detail — and provide a table comparing average blood glucose to A1C — in Chapter 2.

1 Used to Be on Pills, but Now I'm on Insulin. Does that Mean I've Developed Type 1 Diabetes?

No, you still have type 2 diabetes. We can say that you have *insulin-treated* diabetes, but that's not the same as having type 1 diabetes, where you would be absolutely dependent on insulin to stay alive, not just to maintain good blood glucose control.

Once You're on Insulin You're on It Forever, Right?

If you have type 1 diabetes, then yes, you need to be on insulin, and for all intents and purposes it will be forever (or until we have a cure).

If you have type 2 diabetes and, despite appropriate lifestyle and oral hypoglycemic agent therapy, your blood glucose control is still not what it should be, then yes, you really need to be on insulin, and yes, it will likely be forever. But if you're starting out with much to improve in your lifestyle, then there is a significant chance that with diet, exercise, and weight loss, oral hypoglycemic agent therapy will start to work better and, sometimes, effectively enough that you may end up being able to come off insulin.

I'm Watching My Diet, So Why Is My Cholesterol Level High?

Some people can eat a bacon double cheeseburger and have normal cholesterol levels. And other people could order a veggie burger and have abnormal cholesterol levels. The difference? Genetics. Some people are simply genetically programmed to have livers that manufacture excess cholesterol. Indeed, all of us produce the bulk of our cholesterol within our bodies. If you have a body that tends to over-produce cholesterol, you can combat this by following a proper diet, exercising, and getting your blood glucose control in order — but often this is not sufficient. Our genes are very strong. Often that helps us. Sometimes it doesn't.

Why Do I Need Blood Pressure Pills If My Blood Pressure Is Good?

There are two reasons for taking blood pressure medication even when your blood pressure is good:

- ✔ Good blood pressure is seldom good enough.

- ✔ Certain types of blood pressure pills also have other important roles to play that are separate from and independent of their blood pressure–lowering function.

If you have diabetes, then your risk of cardiovascular, kidney, and eye disease is high enough that your blood pressure can't just be good or okay. It has to be perfect. Great. Excellent. Spectacular. Marvellous. Stupendous. . . . Optimal blood pressure will go a lot farther in keeping you healthy than will good blood pressure. And to achieve optimal blood pressure (less than 130/80), high blood pressure medicines are often required.

ACE inhibitors and ARBs are commonly called *blood pressure pills;* however, studies have shown that these medicines do more than just lower blood pressure. Indeed, even if your blood pressure is within target to begin with, these medicines can lower your risk of a heart attack (if you're at high risk) and help prevent deterioration in your kidney function (if you have evidence of kidney damage).

How Can I Get the Most Out of Each Visit to My Doctor?

Congratulations. That you have asked this question tells us that you want to be an active participant in your health care. You aren't content to assume that everything must be okay because your doctor hasn't told you otherwise. You want to know your blood pressure and your cholesterol levels. You want to know your last A1C and whether your eye doctor observed any retinopathy.

Even if he or she does not necessarily always show it, you can be quite confident that your doctor is absolutely thrilled that you're interested enough in your health that you want to be actively involved in your diabetes management.

If you're feeling in the dark, you can follow several steps to obtain more information. We suggest trying these in the order they are listed, proceeding to the next step if the earlier one didn't meet with success:

1. **Let your doctor know you're interested:** Perhaps your doctor simply doesn't realize that you want to know the specifics of your results. Your first step should always be to simply let your physician know that you are keenly interested in your health and would like to know as much as possible about how you're doing. He or she will likely be overjoyed.

2. **Ask specific questions:** "Doctor, what is my blood pressure?" is more likely to get you a specific number than is asking "Doctor, how's my pressure?" which would likely be met with "It's fine."

3. **Ask for copies of your lab results:** You are fully entitled to knowing what your lab results are (heck, it's your blood and urine after all!), and you are similarly entitled to having a copy of them provided to you. Usually, simply discussing your results with your

doctor is sufficient; however, if you feel that this isn't providing you with enough in the way of specifics, then ask your doctor for a photocopy of your results. When you ask for these, make sure you word your request in a non-threatening way; otherwise, your doctor may feel that you are second guessing his or her judgment (which you may be, but there's no benefit to you if your doctor feels defensive). Try something like "Doctor, I like to keep tabs on my lab results. May I please have a photocopy for my records?"

4. **Ask other members of your health care team:** If none of the previous steps has succeeded, try asking other members of your health care team. It may well be that if one of your physicians (say, for example, your diabetes specialist) is not readily forthcoming, another one may be (for example, your family physician). Your diabetes educator is another person to try, because he or she may have received copies of lab results or consultation letters from your physician(s).

Will 1 Always Have Diabetes?

We're sure you can tell why we saved this question for last; it is far and away the most difficult question we ever have to answer. The quick answer is a simple "we don't know" — and, of course, we don't. The more complicated answer is (and this is our personal and highly subjective guess) the following:

✔ If you have type 1 diabetes, you're unlikely to have it forever. It's only a matter of time before a cure is found (perhaps islet cell transplants will get perfected, perhaps gene therapy will be refined, perhaps stem cell research will find an answer, . . .). Sure, you may have heard this prophecy year after year and may be frustrated by the eternal wait. (And who could blame you?) Nonetheless, we can tell you that we would never have used the word *cure* ten years ago, but in the new millennium we dare to mention it. When will a cure be found? That we cannot say. But that there will be one, we have no doubt.

✔ If you have type 2 diabetes, the situation is much trickier, and we suspect that there won't be a cure in the foreseeable future. The factors leading to type 2 diabetes are complex and far from completely understood. It's highly unlikely that we're dealing with a single cause for which there will be a single cure. On the other hand, more and better treatment options are rapidly emerging. Even if we can't undo your diabetes, it's likely that we'll be able to offer such effective therapy that your diabetes will become less and less difficult for you to deal with.

As diabetes specialists, we're always full of hope. Every day, research comes out revealing new insights into the condition. And the pace at which new and better therapies are emerging is simply astounding. The single greatest advantage to you in having a disease that's rapidly becoming more common is that this stimulates research scientists to put tremendous resources into finding ways to help you.

When we look back at our careers and see what medical science knows now that it did not when we first began our practices, we can only marvel at the progress we've made in our quest to keep people with diabetes healthy. Some people with diabetes, alas, tell us they do not feel that scientists are really looking for a cure. We find this comment so sad, for it is so untrue. Thousands of scientists — people who have dedicated their entire careers to this cause — are looking for a cure. Not just finding a new, expensive drug to control diabetes, but an honest-to-goodness cure. How can we be so certain? Because we read their research papers, and hear them speak, and meet them all the time.

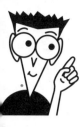

Making everything easier!

HEALTH AND SELF HELP

Breast Cancer For Dummies
978-07645-2482-0

Celiac Disease For Dummies
978-0-470-16036-7

Cognitive Behavioral Therapy For Dummies
978-0-470-01838-5

Diabetes Cookbook For Canadians For Dummies, 1st Edition
978-0-470-16028-2

Diabetes For Canadians For Dummies, 2nd Edition
978-0-470-15677-3

Emotional Intelligence For Dummies
978-0-470-15732-9

Nutrition For Canadians For Dummies
978-0-470-15307-9

Understanding Prescription Drugs For Canadians For Dummies
978-0-470-83835-8

Understanding Autism For Dummies
978-0-7645-2547-6

FOOD, HOME & MUSIC

30-Minute Meals For Dummies
978-0-7645-2589-6

Canadian Wine For Dummies
978-1-894413-18-3

Flipping Houses For Canadians For Dummies
978-0-470-15733-6

Gluten-Free Cooking For Dummies
978-0-470-17810-2

Guitar For Dummies 2e
978-0-7645-9904-0

Home Winemaking For Dummies
978-0-470-67895-4

Organizing For Dummies
978-0-470-43111-5

Trumpet For Dummies
978-0-470-67937-1

Violin For Dummies
978-0-470-83838-9

EDUCATION

Algebra For Dummies, 2nd Edition
978-0-470-55964-2

Calculus For Dummies
978-0-7645-2498-1

Canadian History for Dummies 2nd Edition
978-0-470-83656-9

English Grammar For Dummies
978-0-470-54664-2

Spanish For Dummies
978-0-470-46244-7

Sports Psychology For Dummies
978-0-470-67659-2

Statistics For Dummies
978-0-7645-5423-0

The Canadian GED For Dummies
978-0-470-68091-9

World History For Dummies
978-0-470-44654-6

COMPUTERS & DIGITAL MEDIA

Canon EOS Rebel T2i/550D For Dummies
978-0-470-76881-5

Digital Photography For Dummies
978-0-470-25074-7

iPad™ Portable Genius
978-0-470-54096-1

iPhone For Dummies, 4th Edition
978-0-470-87870-5

Microsoft Excel 2010 For Dummies
978-0-470-48953-6

Microsoft Office 2010 For Dummies
978-0-470-48998-7

Mac OS X Snow Leopard For Dummies
978-0-470-43543-4

Windows 7 For Dummies
978-0-470-49743-2

Windows 7 For Seniors For Dummies
978-0-470-50946-3

Available wherever books are sold.
Go to www.dummies.com or call 1-800-567-4797 to order direct

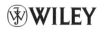

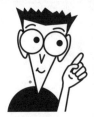

The easy way to get more done and have more fun!

PERSONAL FINANCE & BUSINESS

78 Tax Tips For Canadians
For Dummies
978-0-470-67658-5

Accounting For Canadians
For Dummies
978-0-470-83878-5

Bookkeeping For Canadians
For Dummies
978-0-470-73762-0

Buying & Selling a Home For
Canadians For Dummies, 4th Edition
978-0470-96402-6

Day Trading For Canadians
For Dummies
978-0-470-94503-2

Canadian Small Business Kit
For Dummies, 3rd Edition
978-0-470-93652-8

Investing For Canadians
For Dummies
978-0-470-16029-9

Personal Finance For Canadians
For Dummies
978-0-470-67988-3

Trading For Canadians
For Dummies
978-0-470-67744-5

FITNESS, HOBBIES & PETS

Curling For Dummies
978-0-470-83828-0

Dog Training For Dummies
2nd Edition
978-0-764-58418-3

Golden Retrievers For Dummies
978-0-7645-5267-0

Golf For Dummies, 3rd Edition
978-0-471-76871-5

Horses For Dummies
978-0-7645-9797-8

Knitting For Dummies
2nd Edition
978-0-470-28747-7

Lacrosse For Dummies
978-0-470-73855-9

Quilting For Dummies
978-0-7645-9799-2

Sewing For Dummies
978-0-7645-6847-3

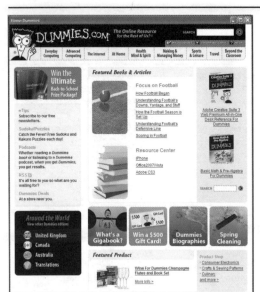

Get smart @ dummies.com®

- Find a full list of Dummies titles
- Look into loads of FREE on-site articles
- Sign up for FREE eTips e-mailed to you weekly
- See what other products carry the Dummies name
- Shop directly from the Dummies bookstore
- Enter to win new prizes every month!

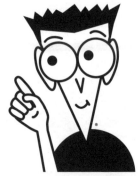

Available wherever books are sold.
Go to www.dummies.com or call 1-800-567-4797 to order direct